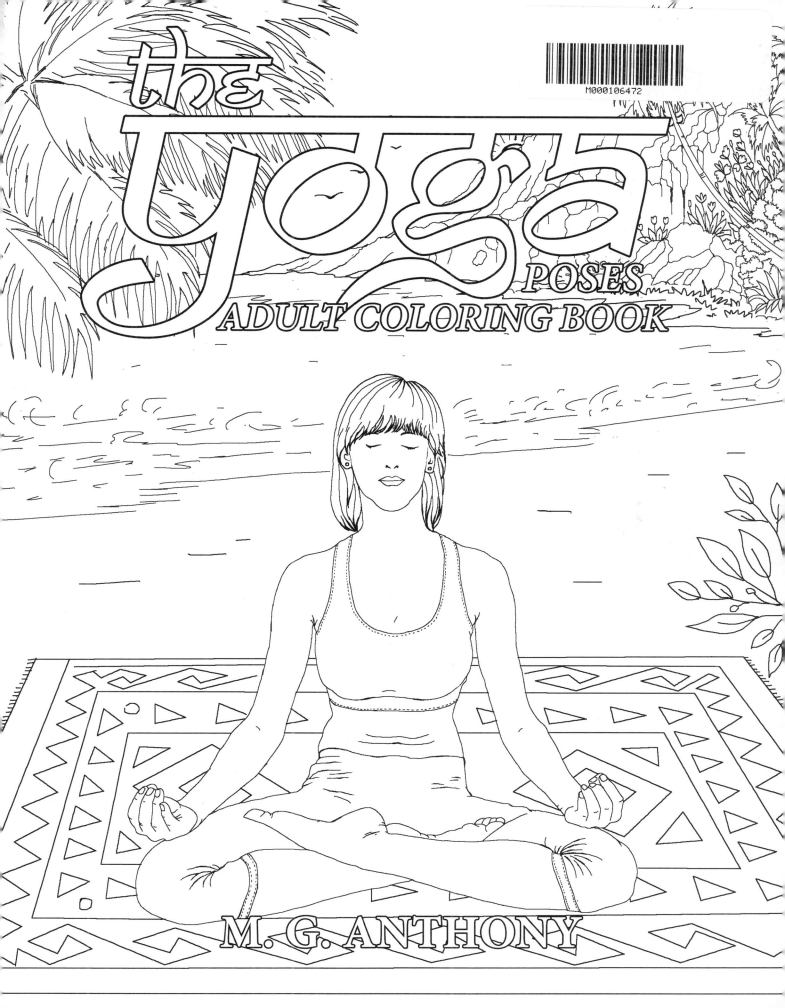

A POST HILL PRESS BOOK

THE YOGA POSES ADULT COLORING BOOK
© 2016 by M. G. Anthony
All Rights Reserved

The book was developed in consultation with the Warwick Yoga Center.
Visit warwickyogacenter.com

The publisher gratefully acknowledges J. Friedman for his contribution to this book.
Namaste.

ISBN: 978-1-68261-130-2

Interior Design and Composition by Greg Johnson, Textbook Perfect

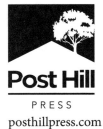

Post Hill
PRESS
posthillpress.com

Printed in the United States of America

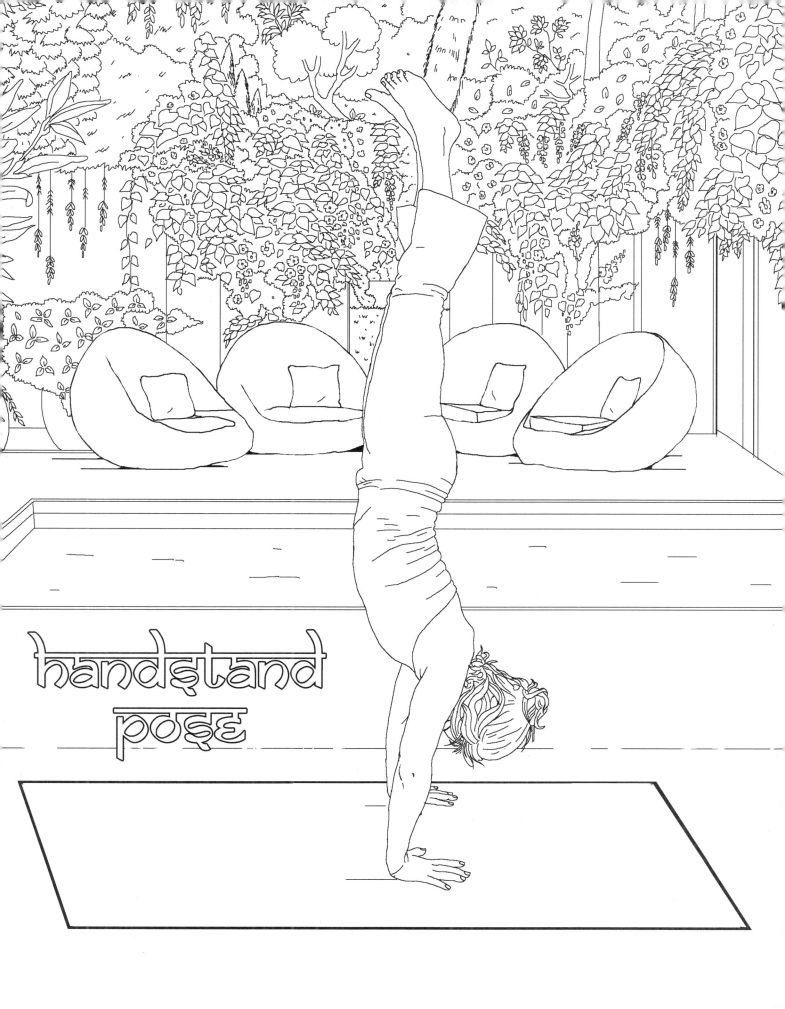

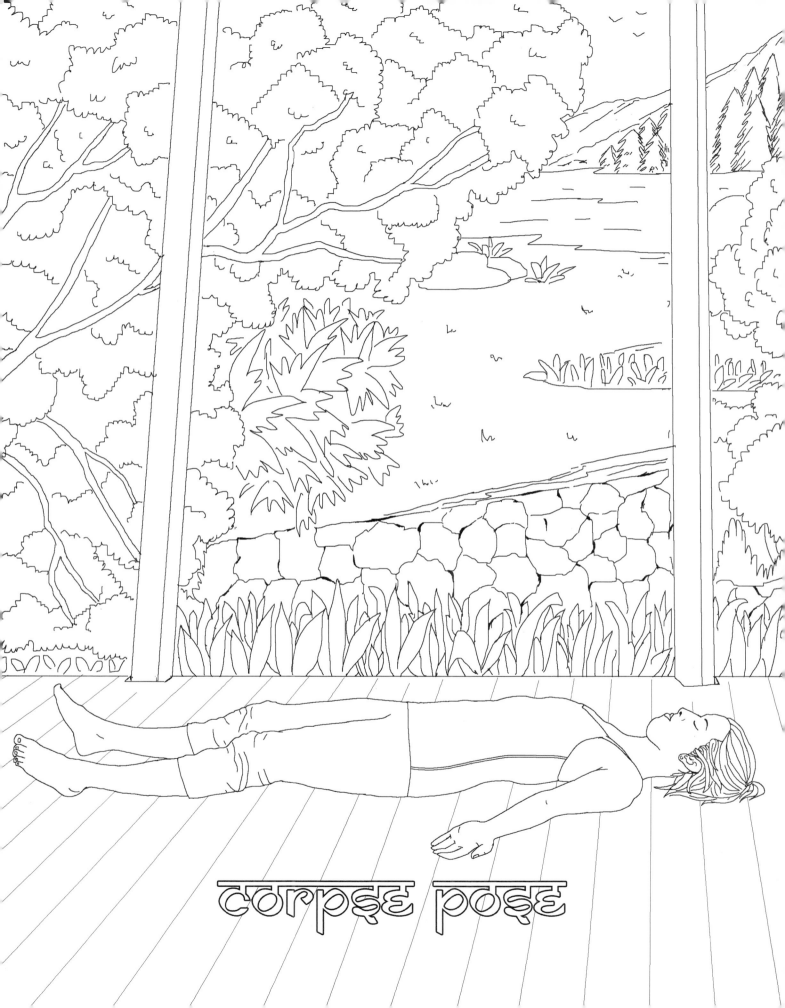

corpse pose

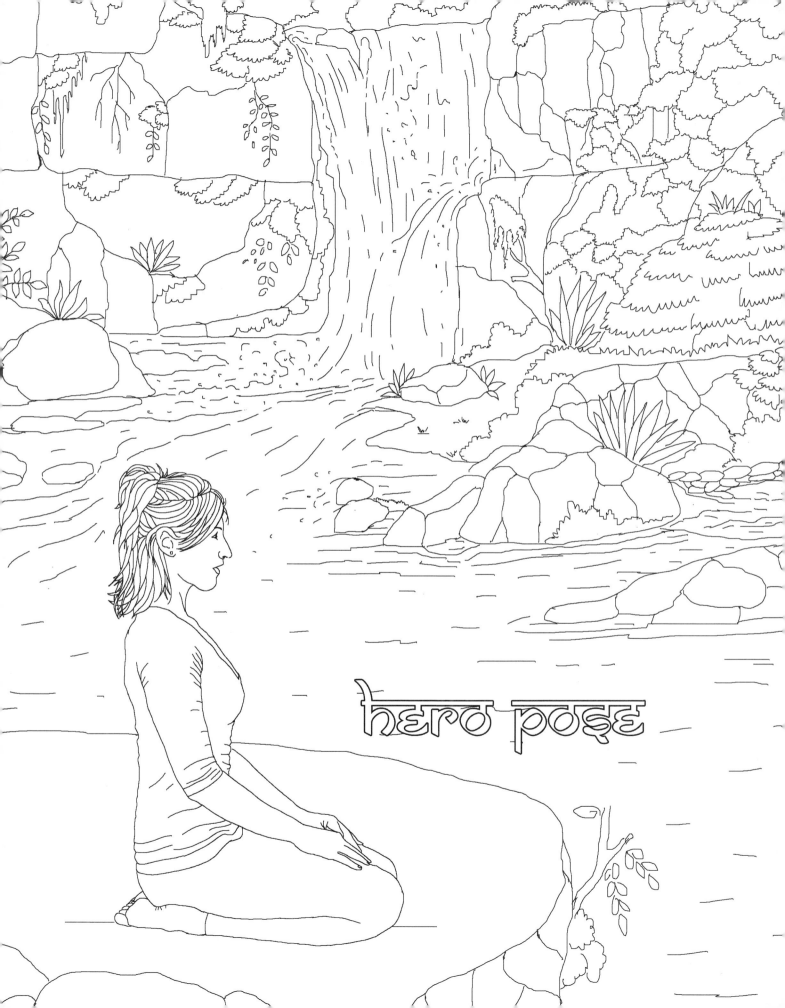

hero pose

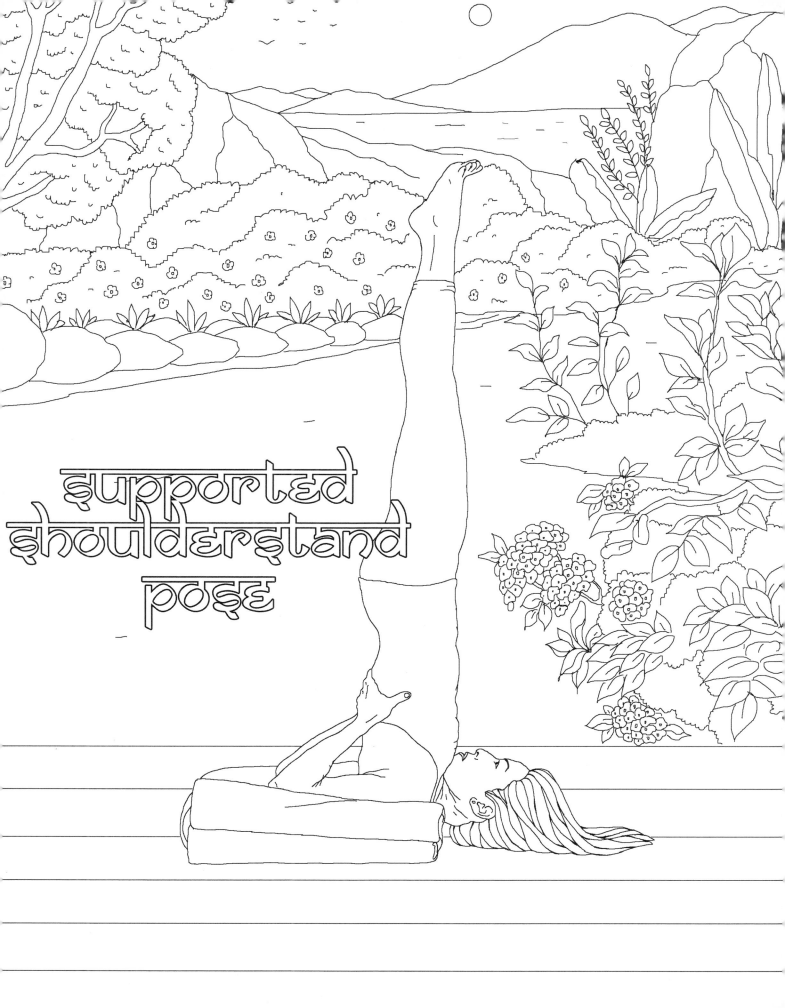

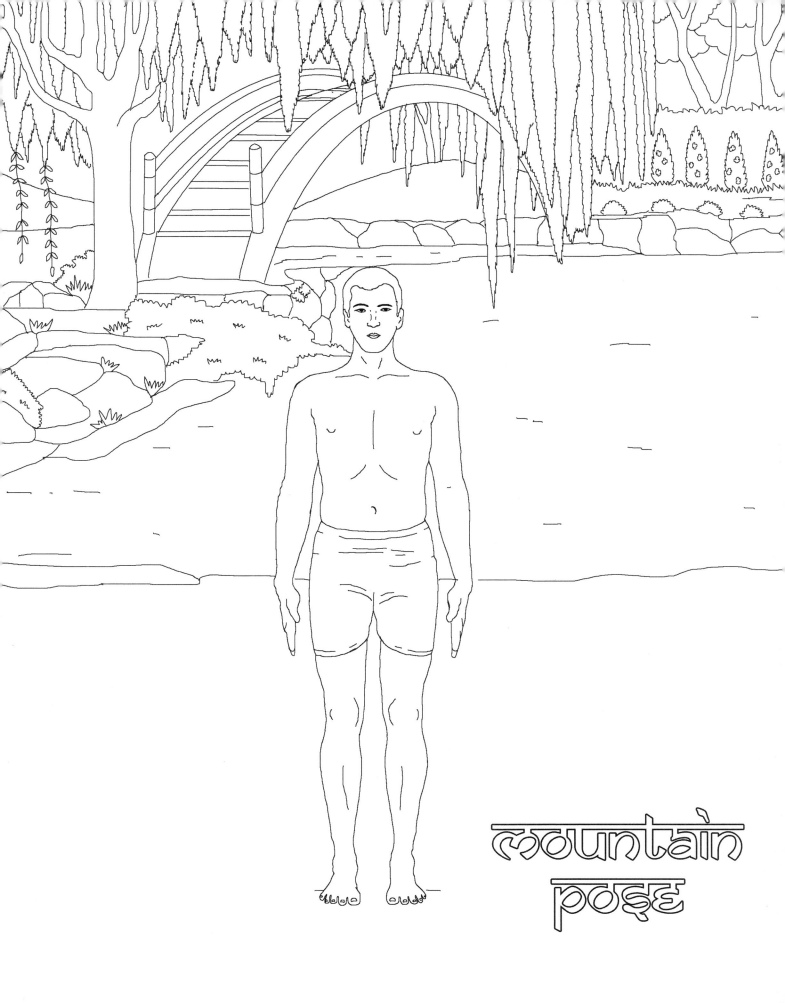

mountain
pose

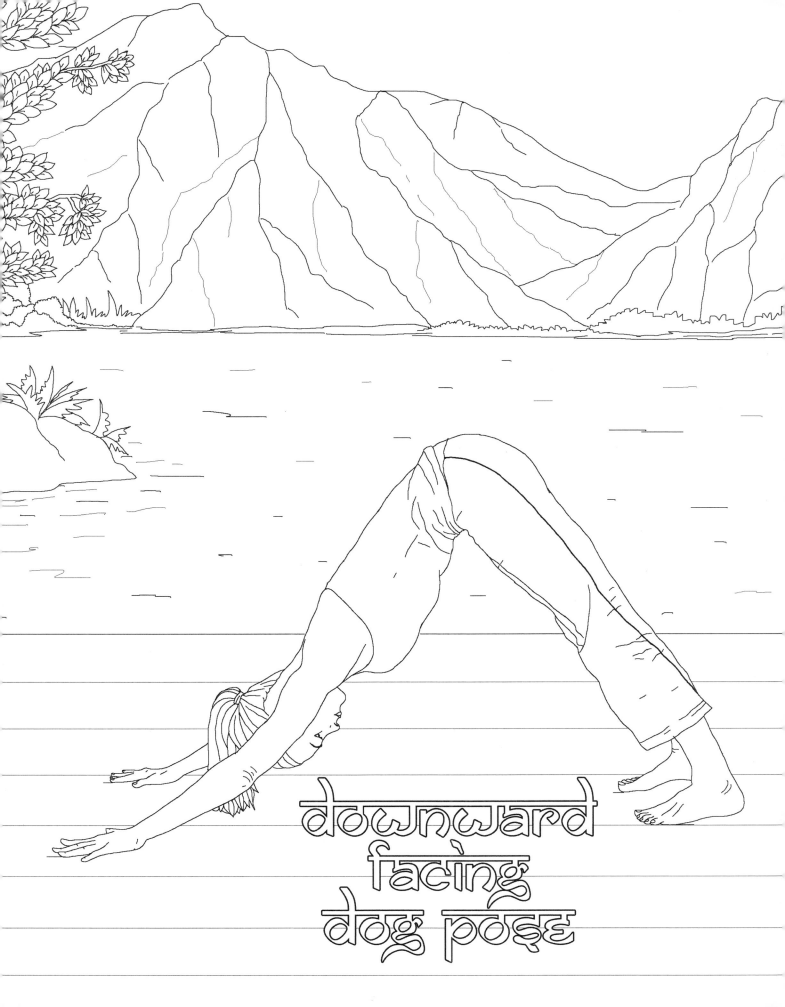

downward
facing
dog pose

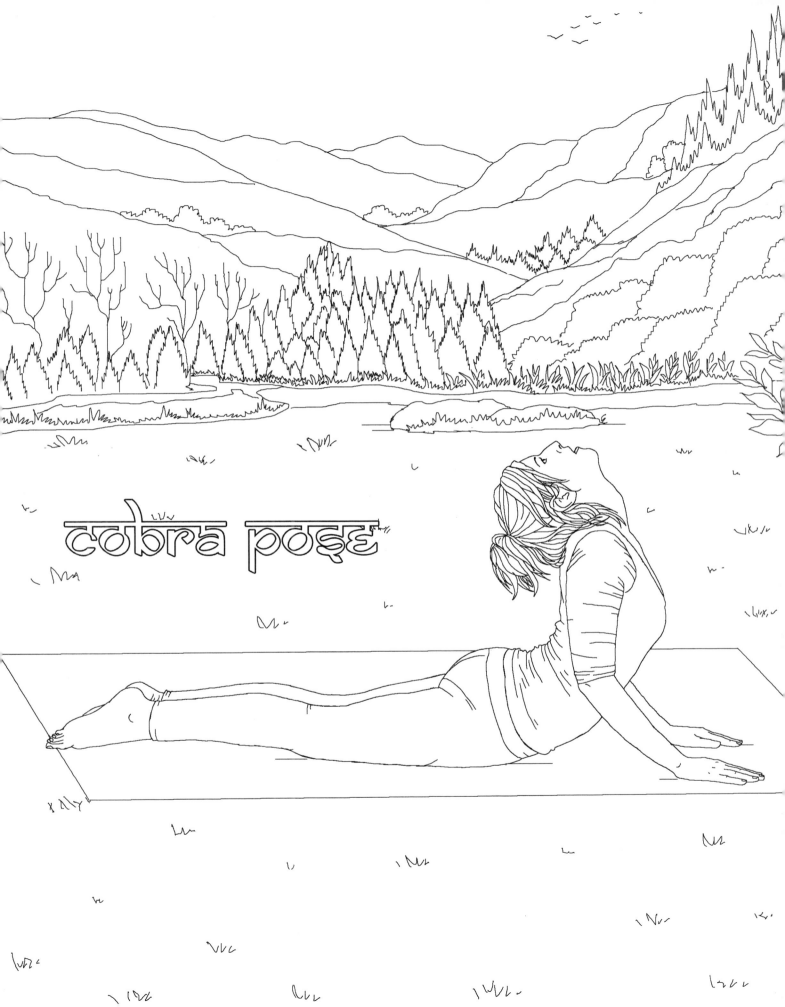

cobra pose

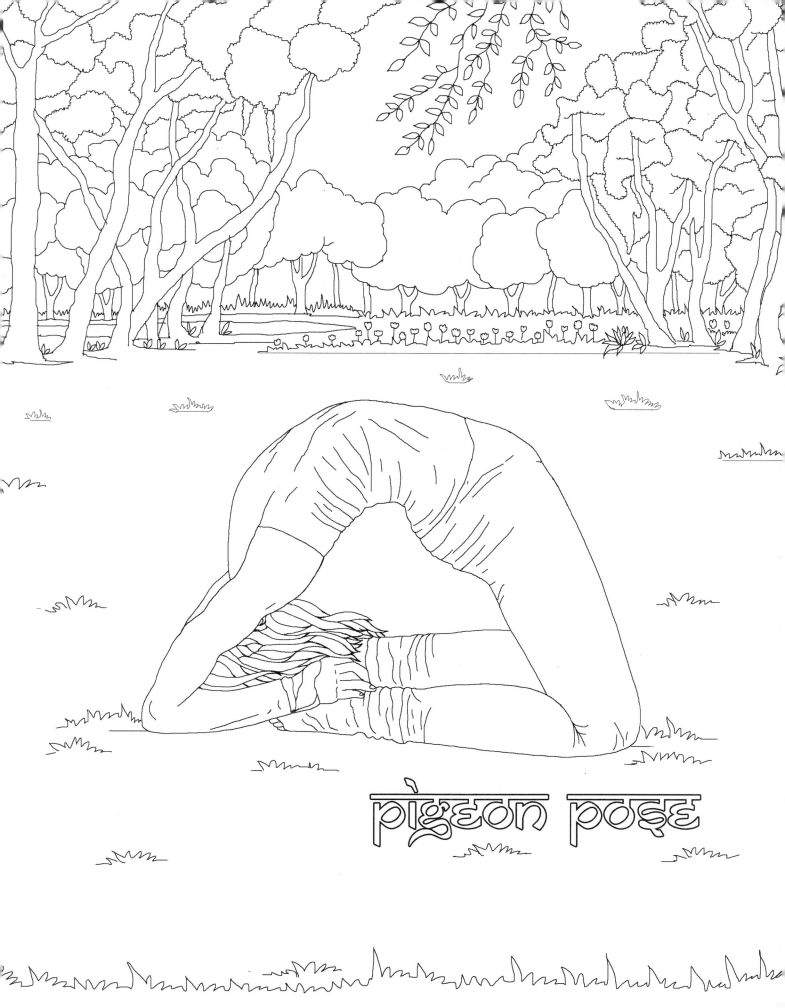

pigeon pose

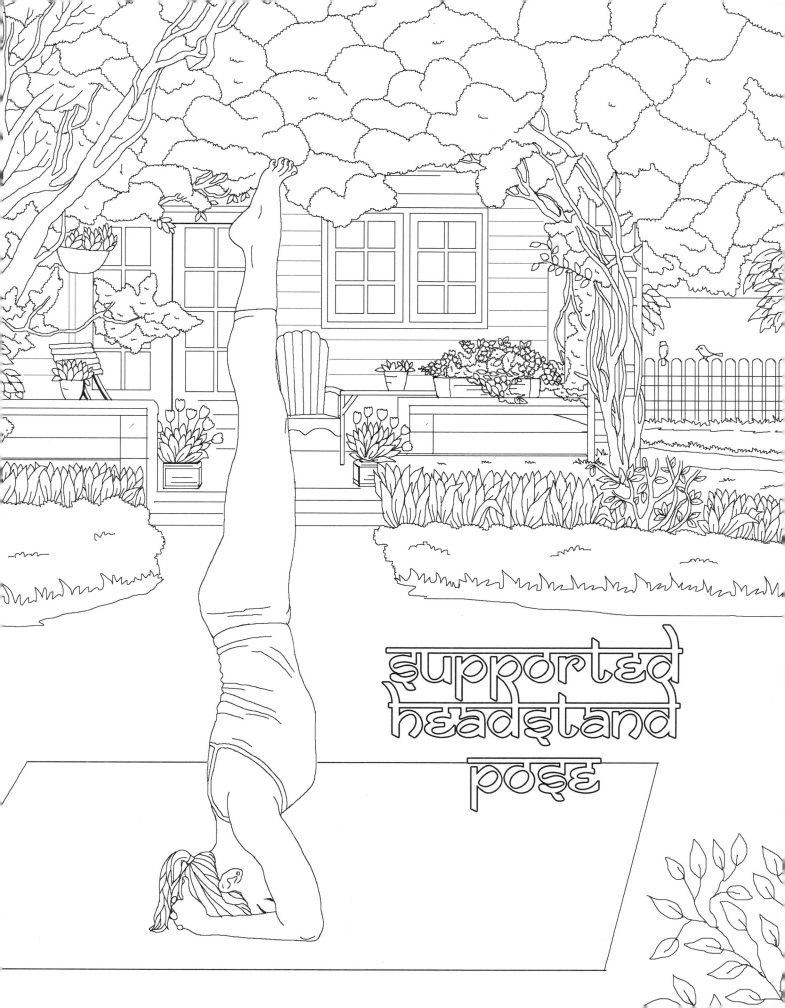

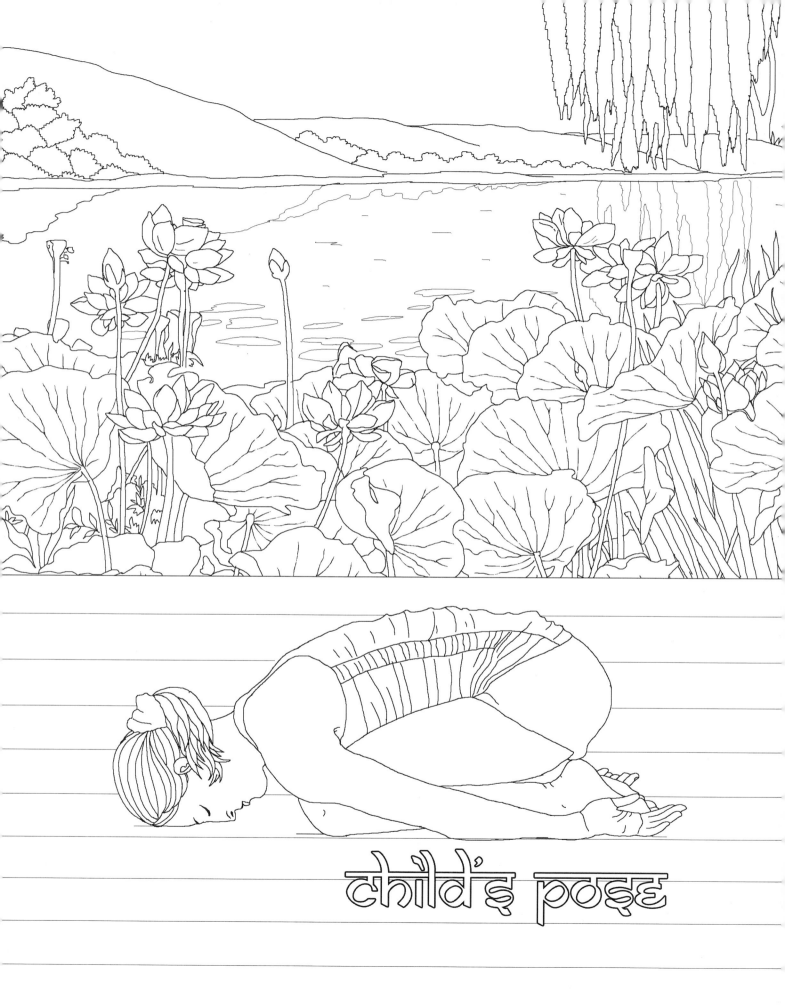

child's pose

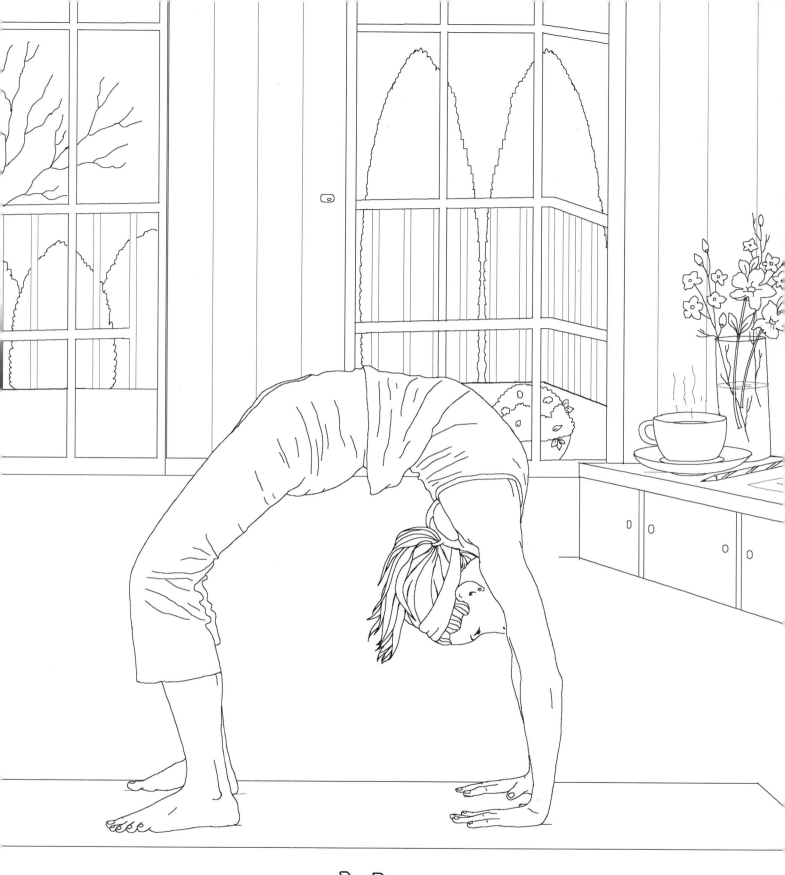

upward bow pose

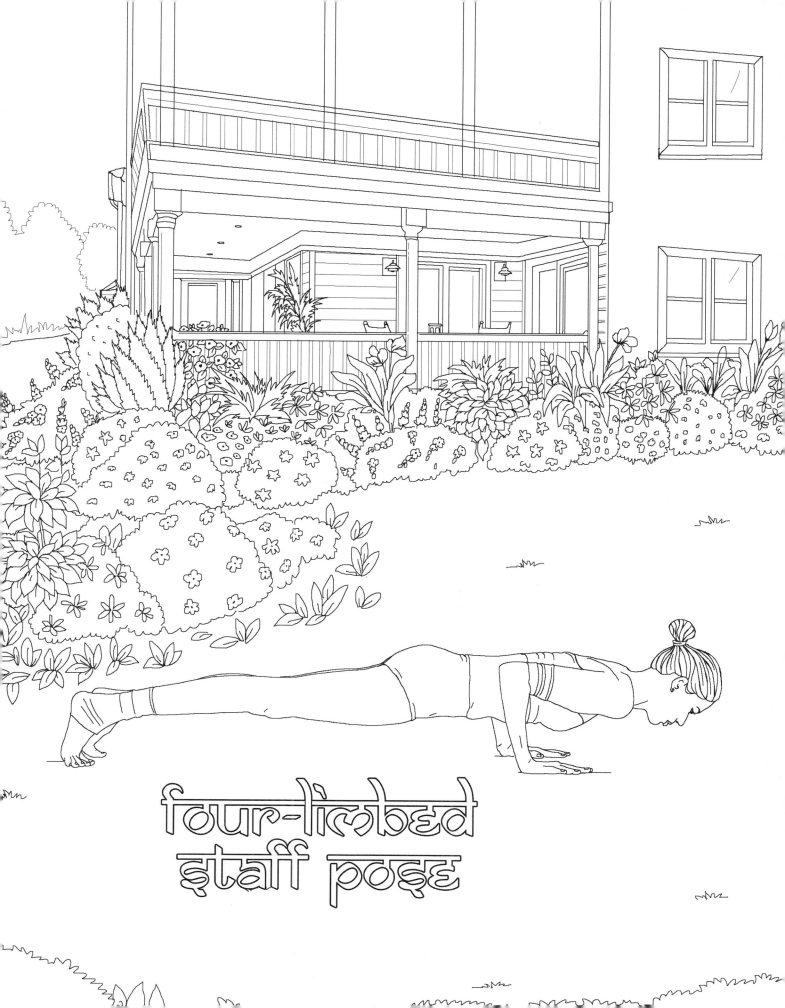

four-limbed
staff pose

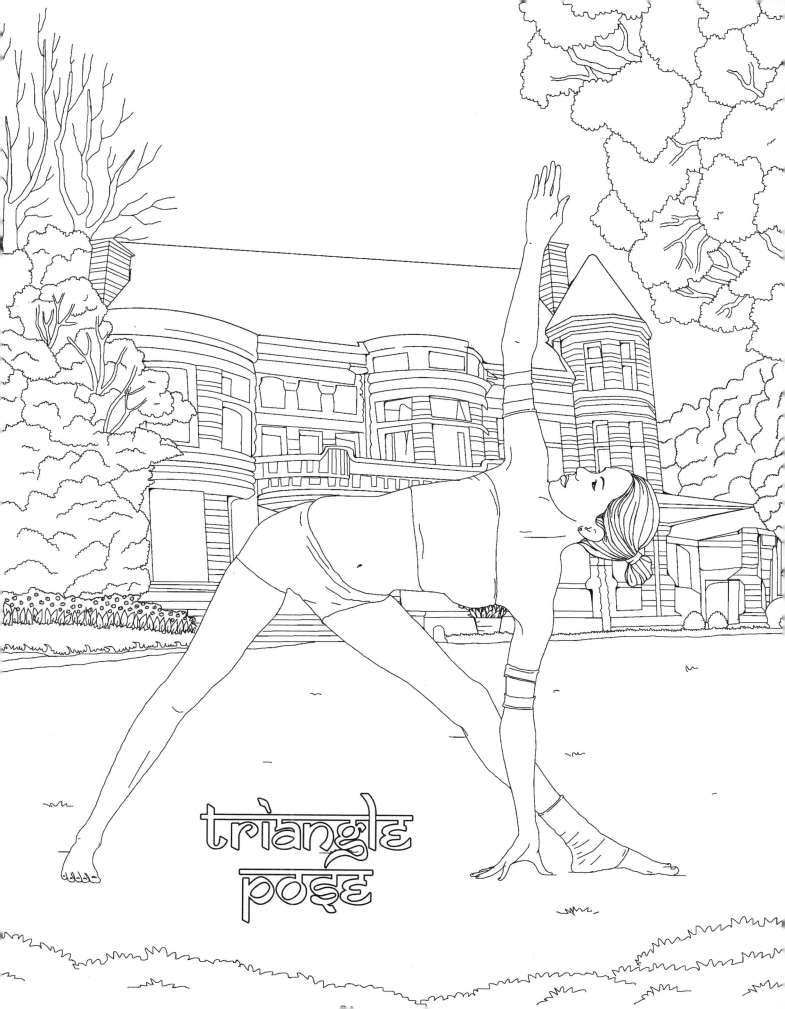

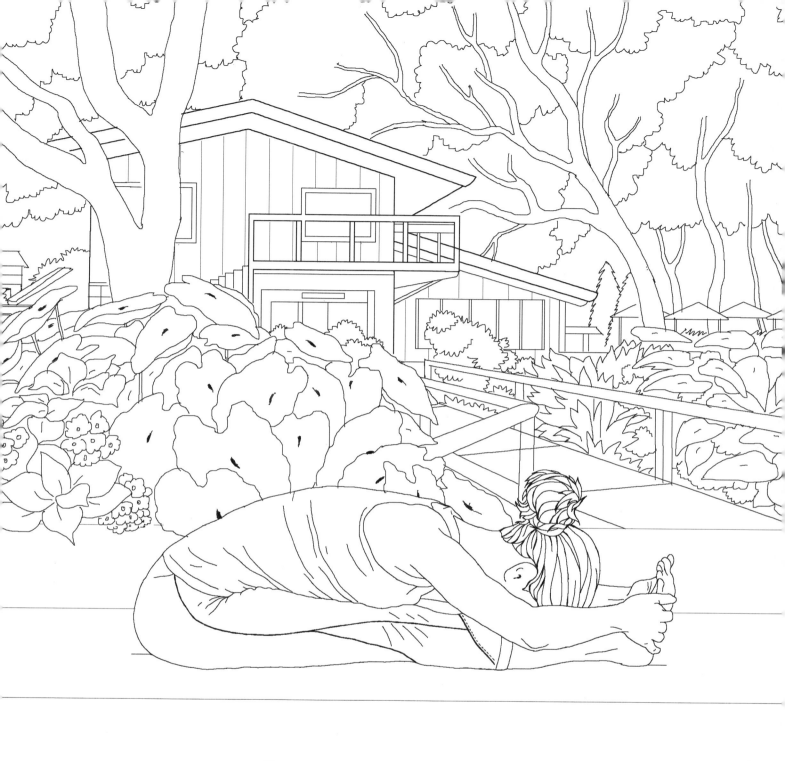

seated forward bend
pose

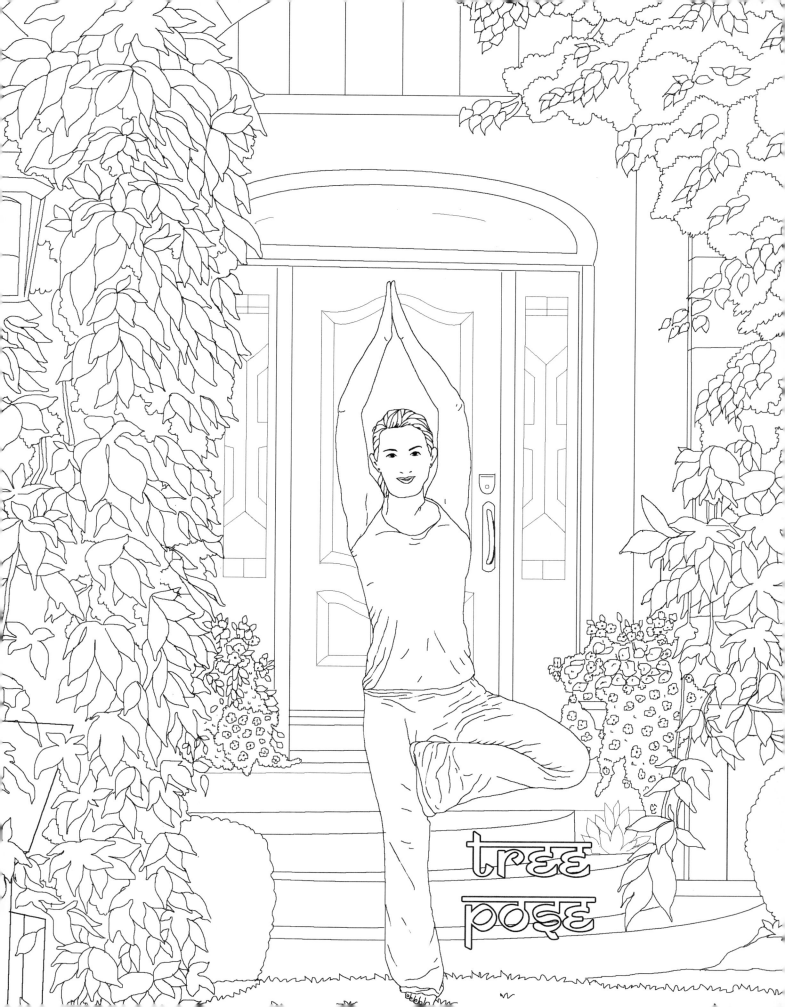

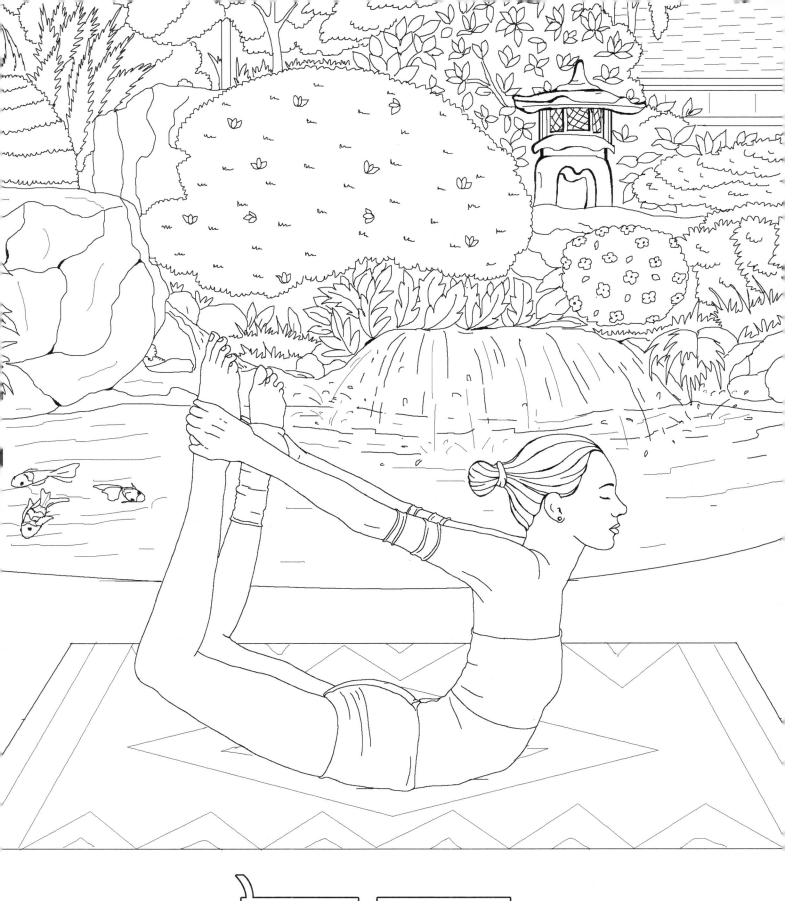

bow pose

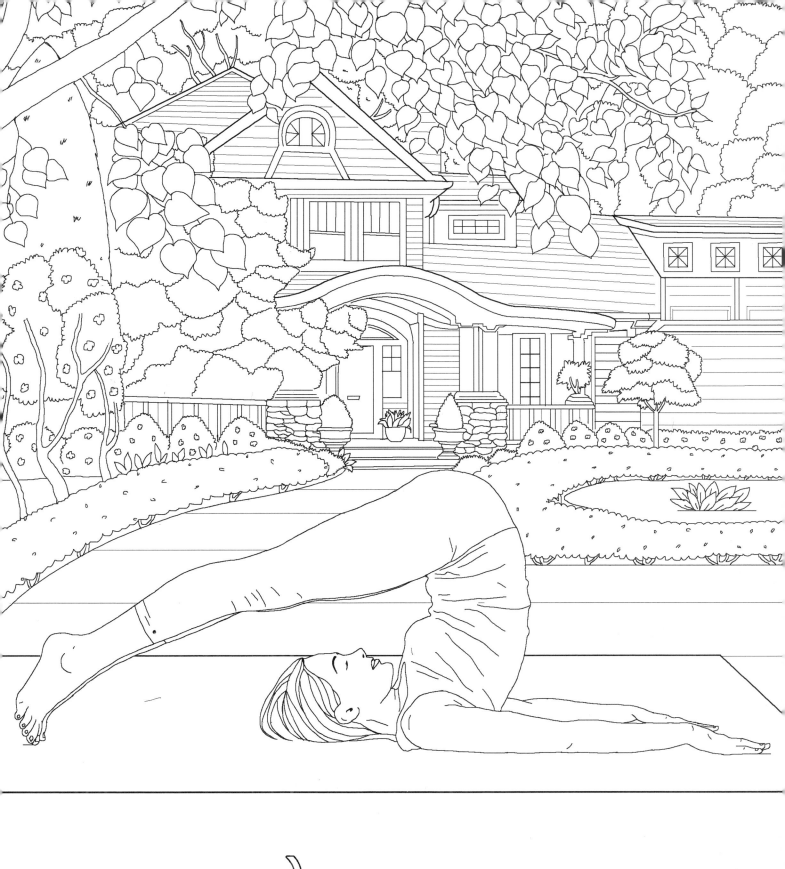

plow pose

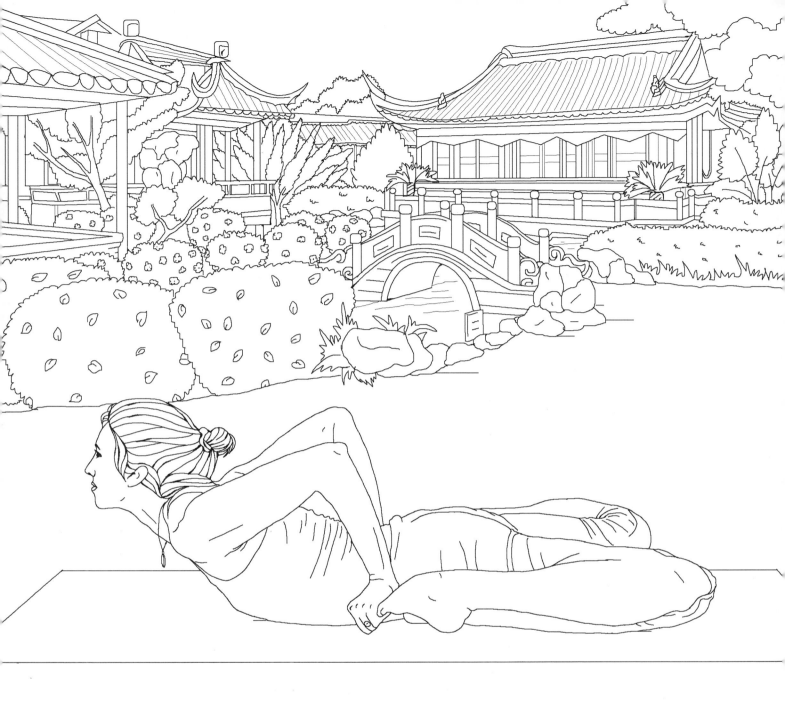

frog pose

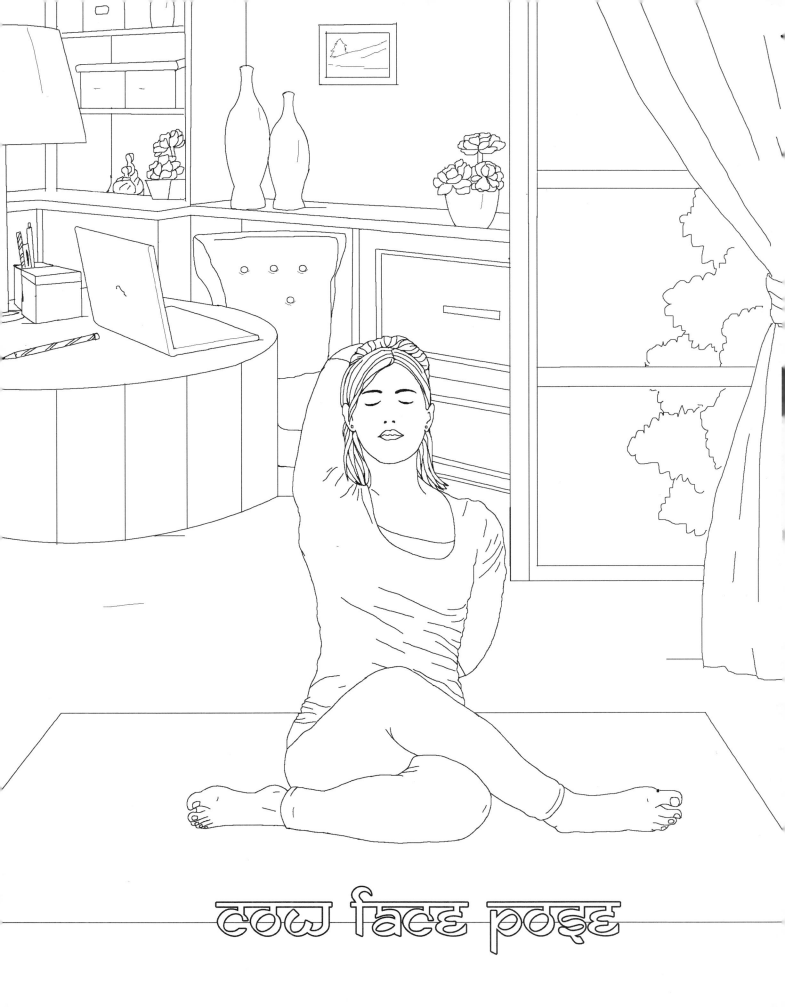

cow face pose

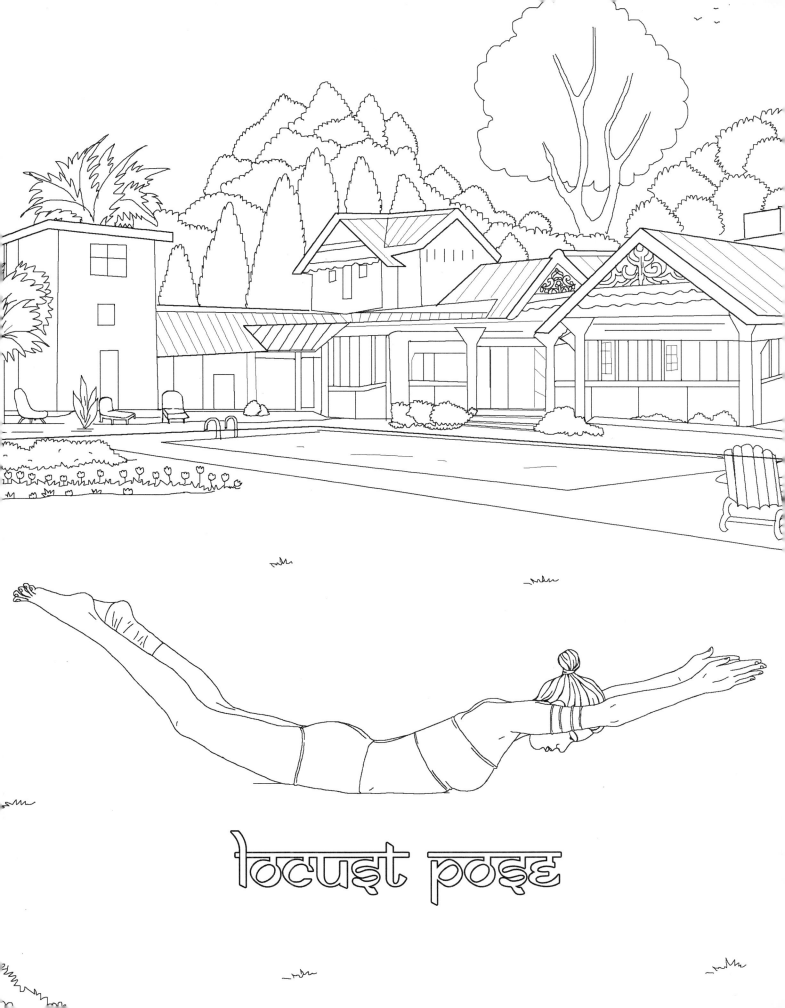

locust pose

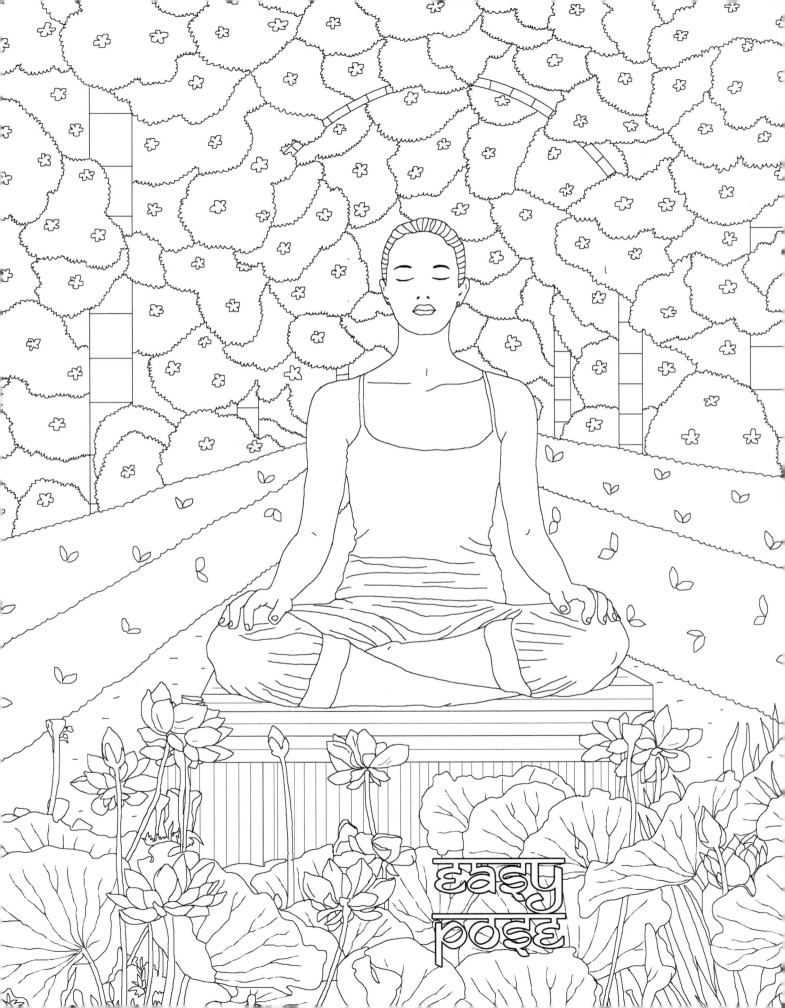

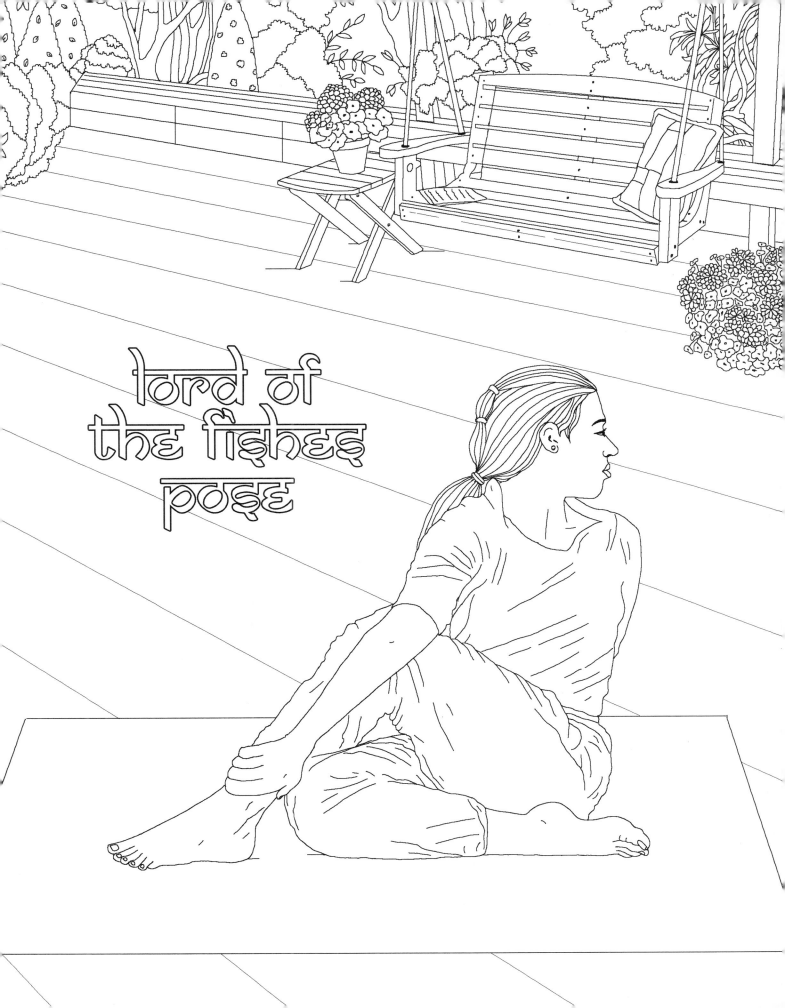

lord of
the fishes
pose

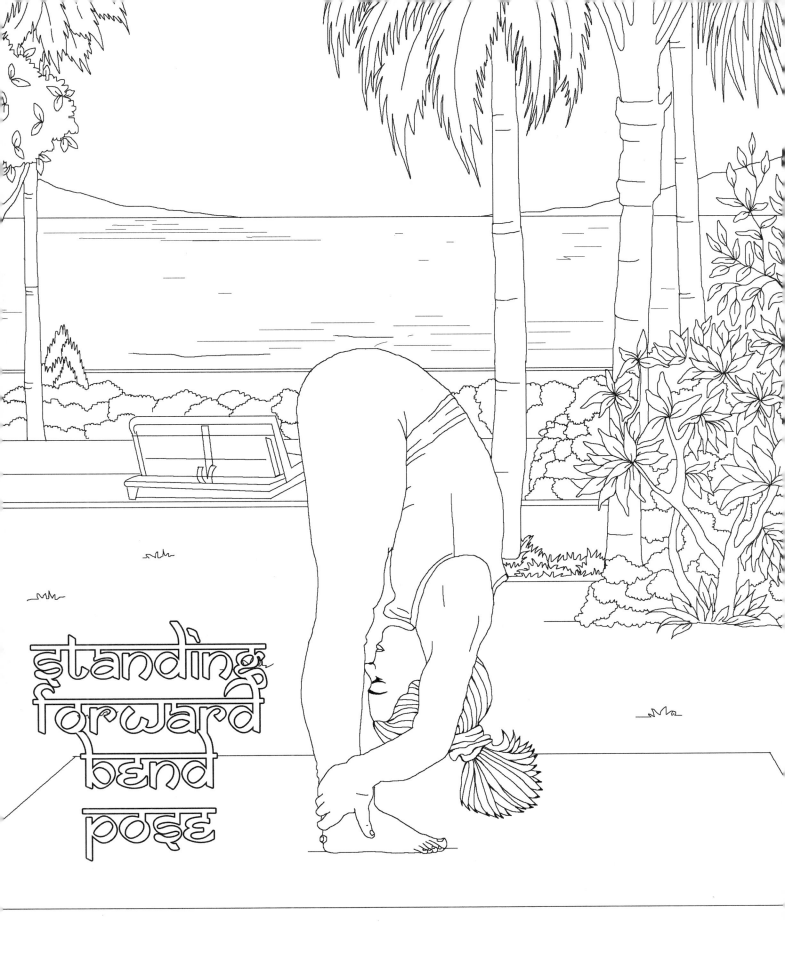

standing forward bend pose

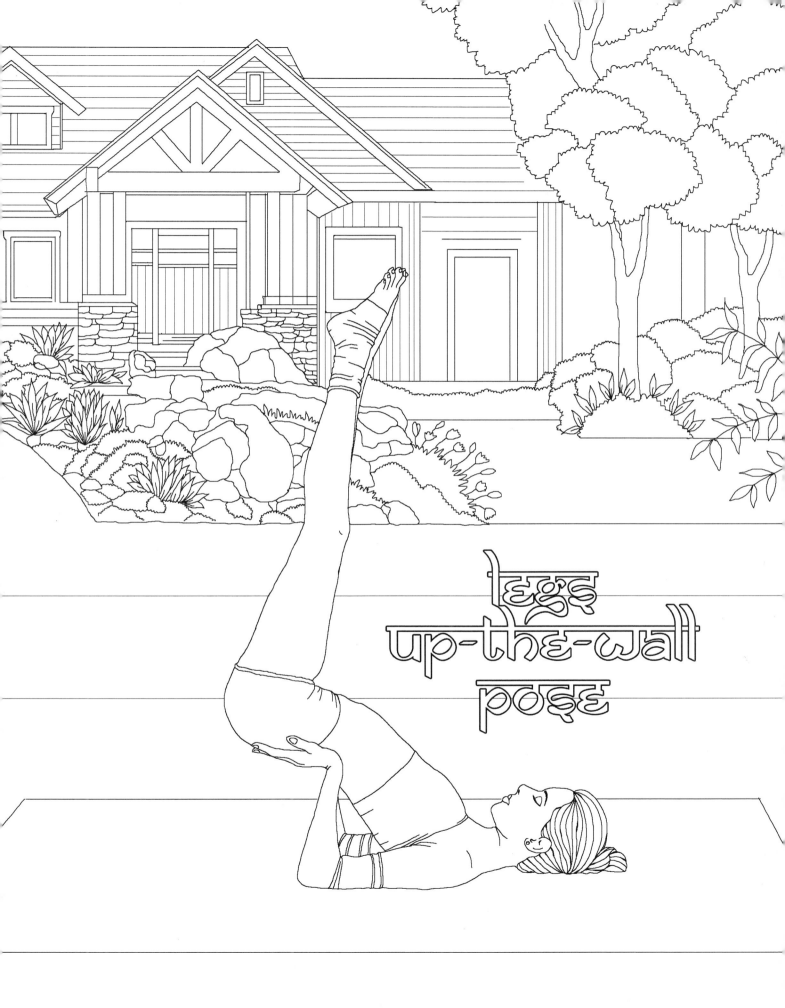

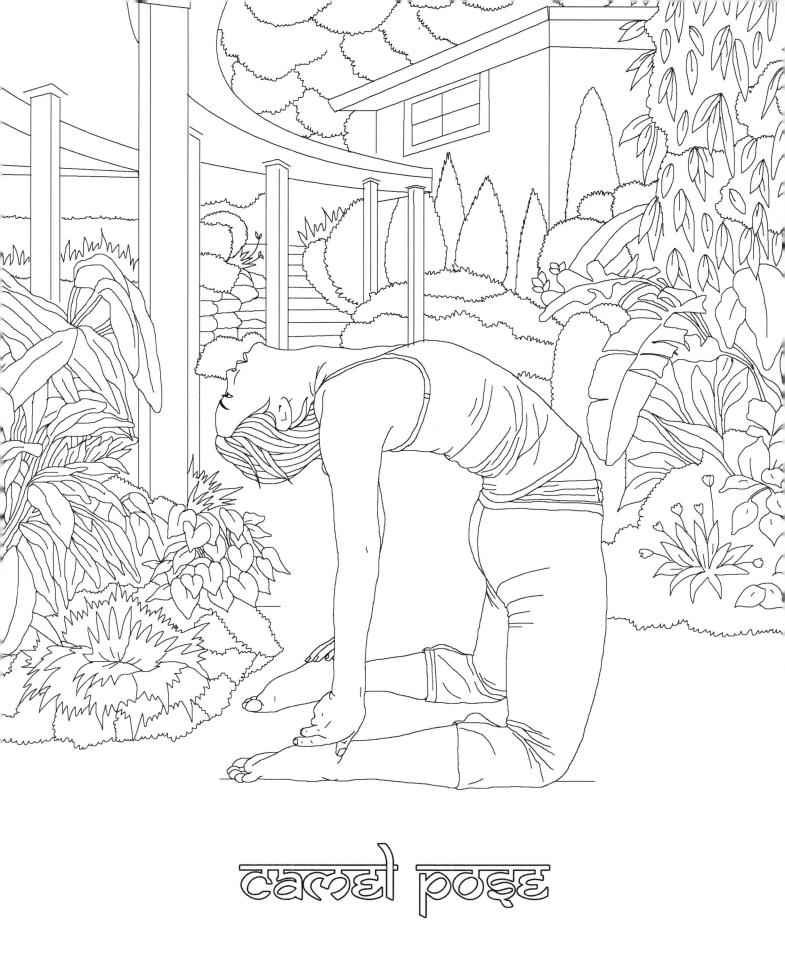

camel pose

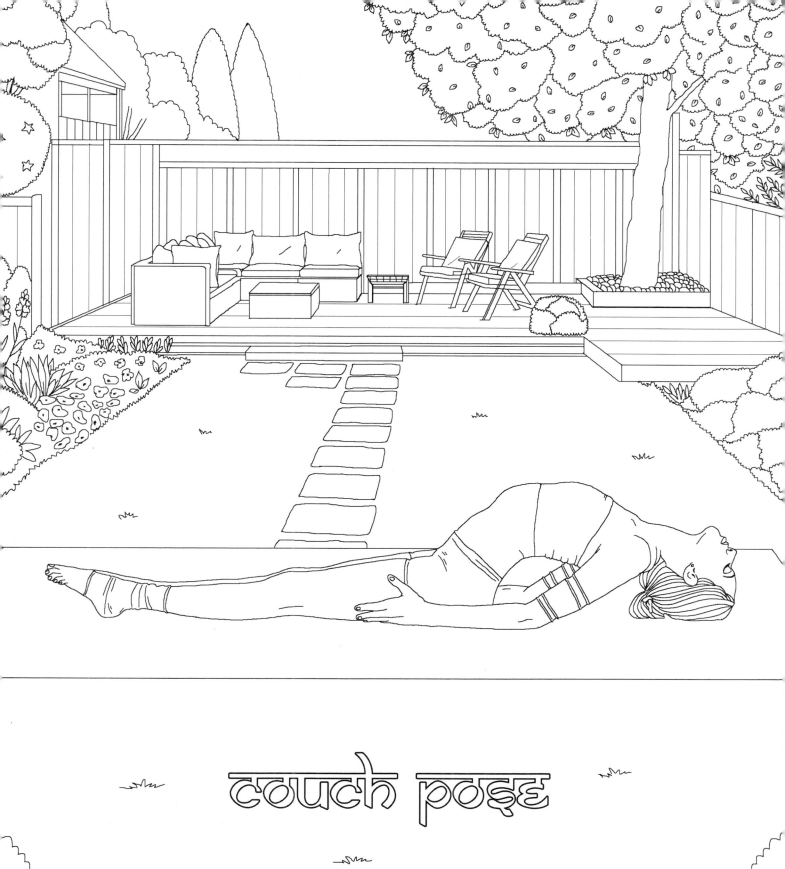

couch pose

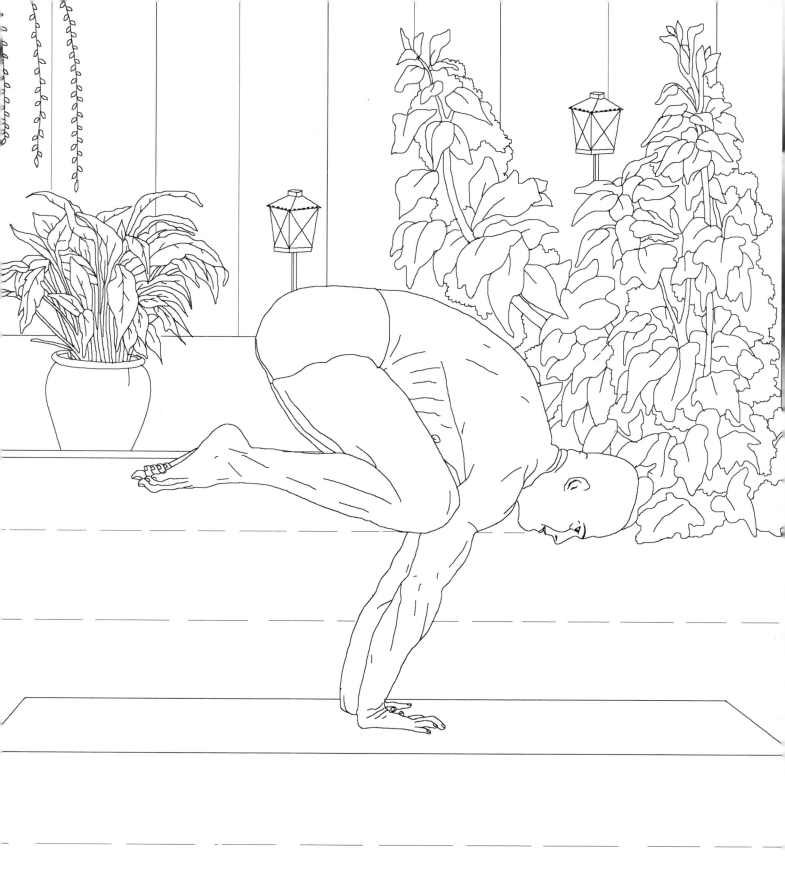

CRANE POSE

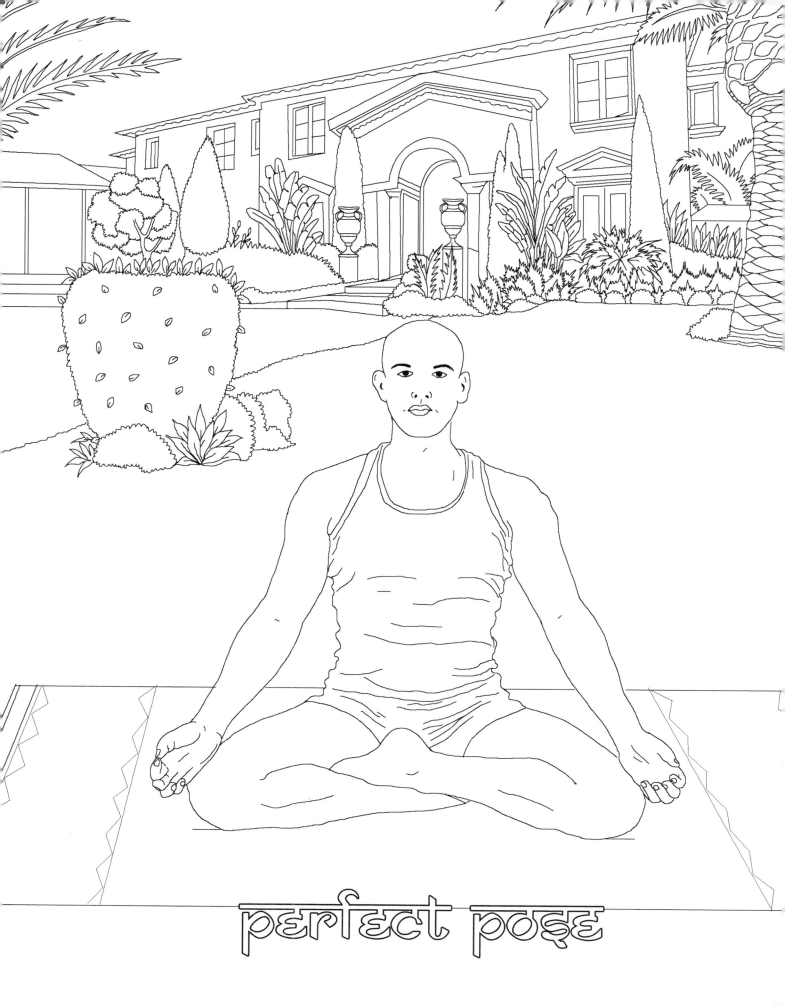

perfect pose

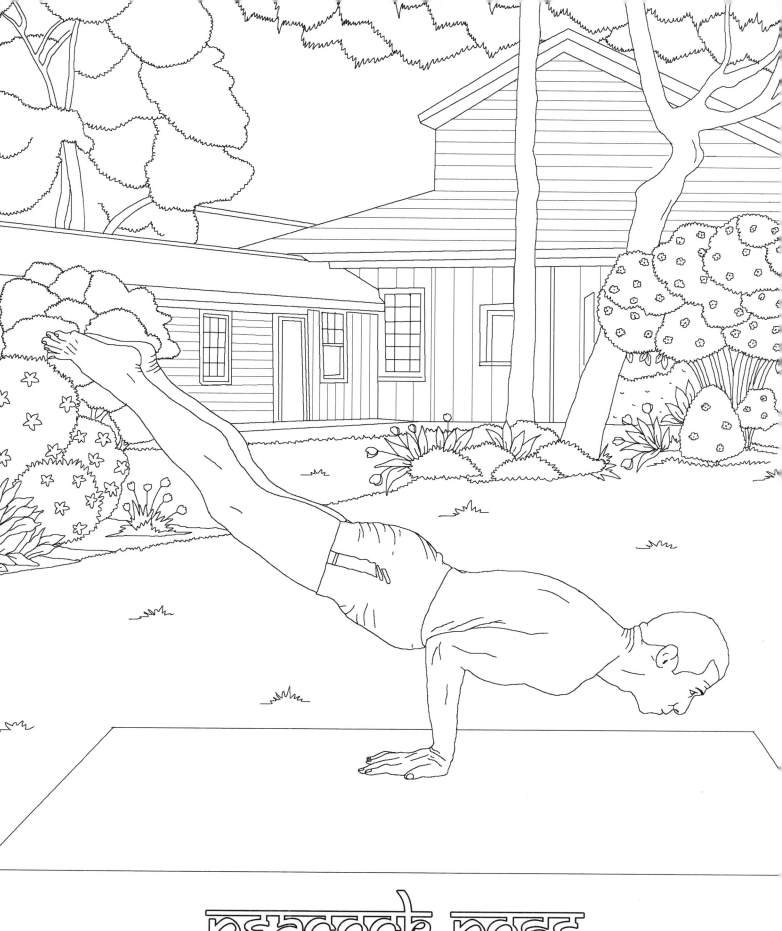

peacock pose

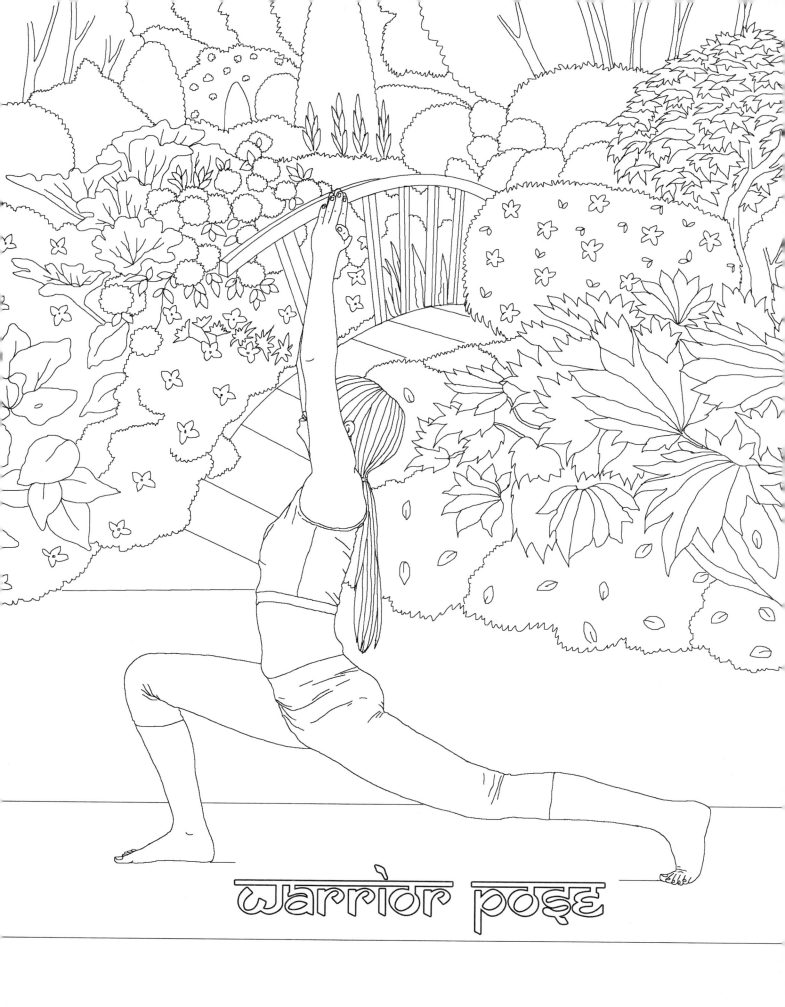

WARRIOR POSE

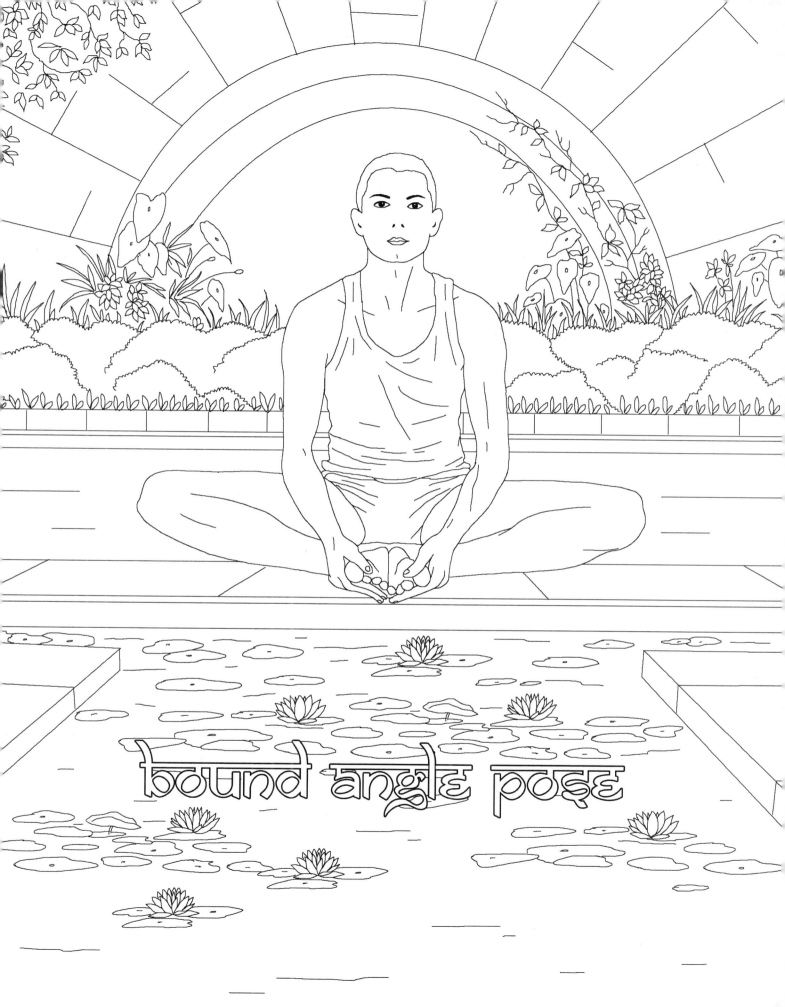

bound angle pose

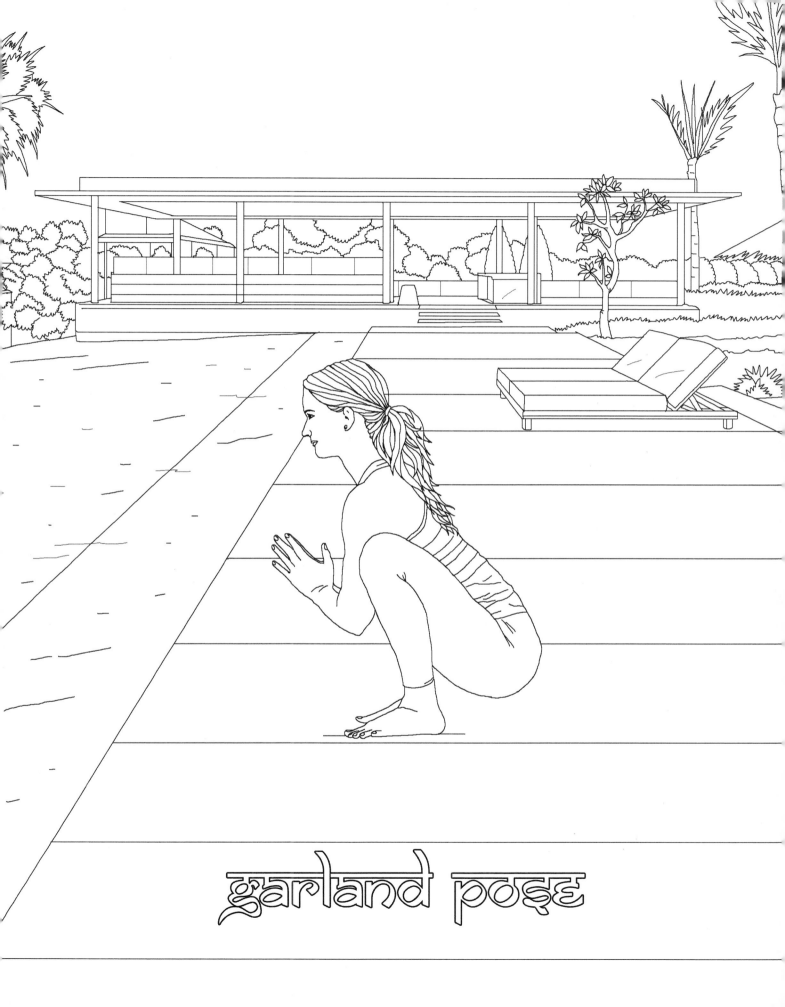

garland pose

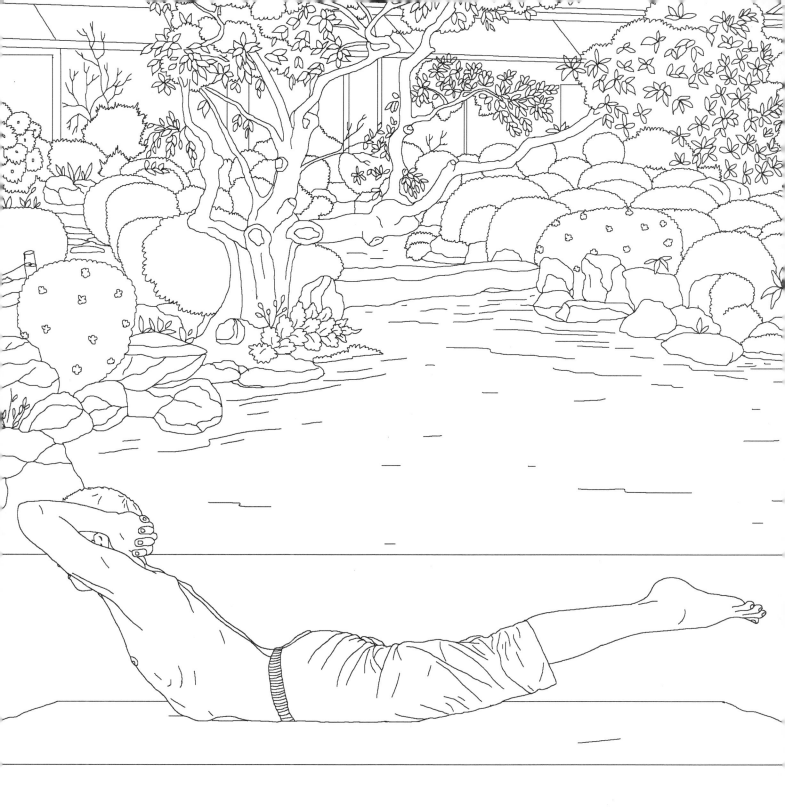

crocodile pose

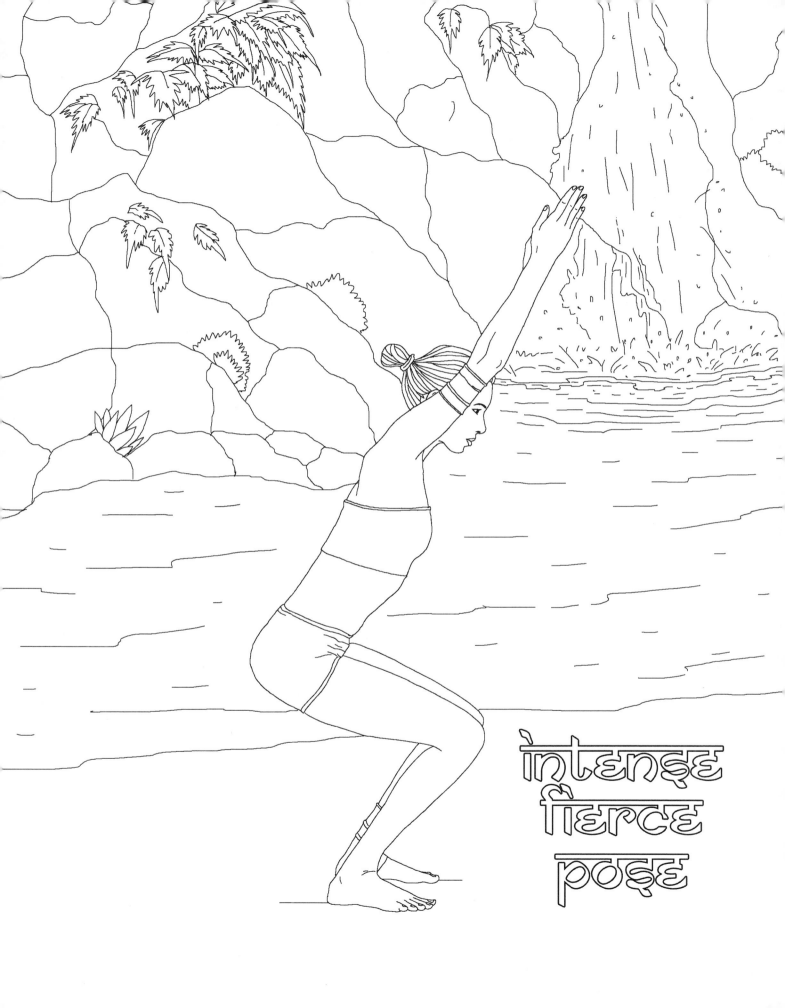

intense fierce pose

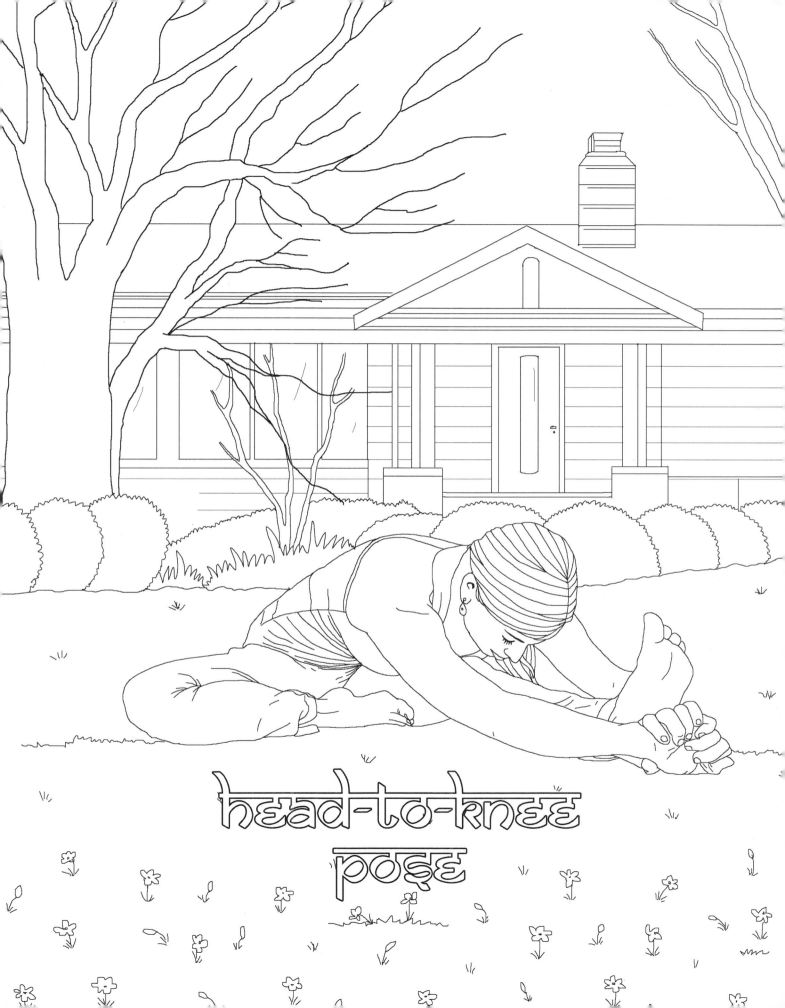

head-to-knee
pose

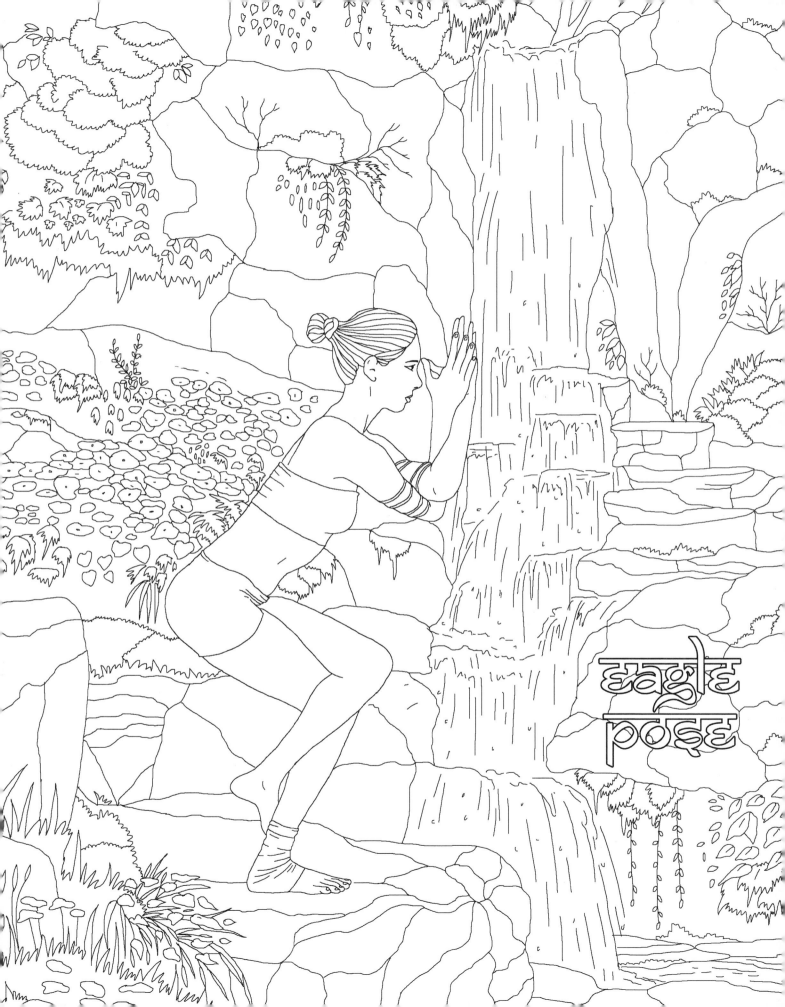

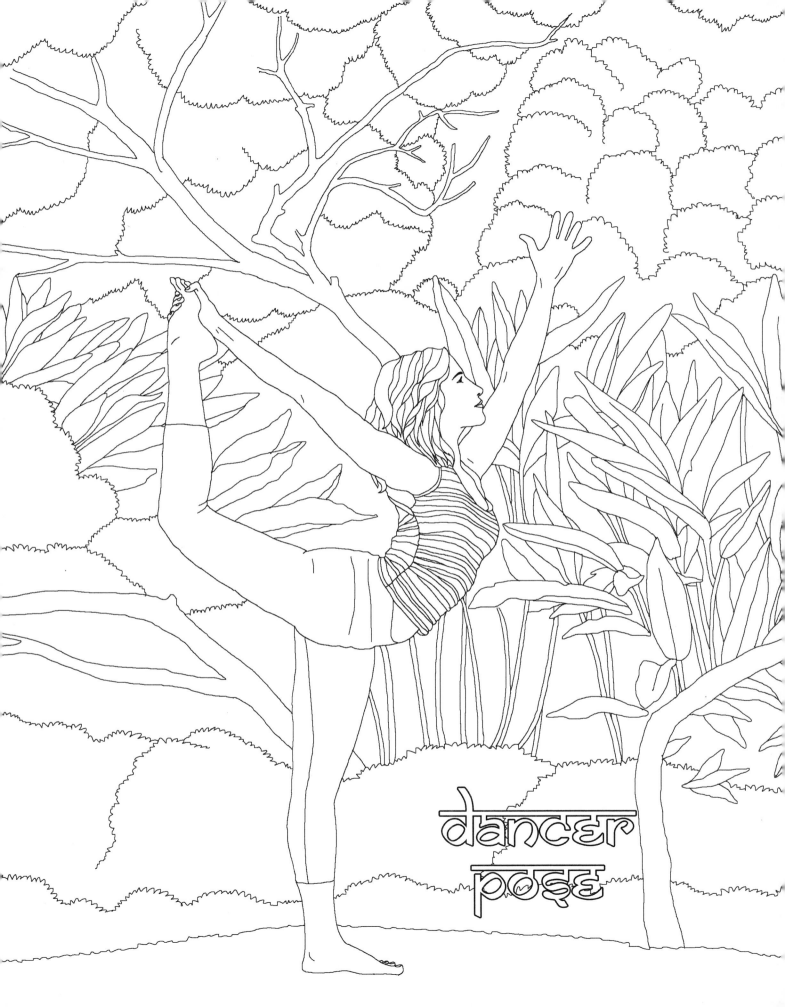

dancer pose

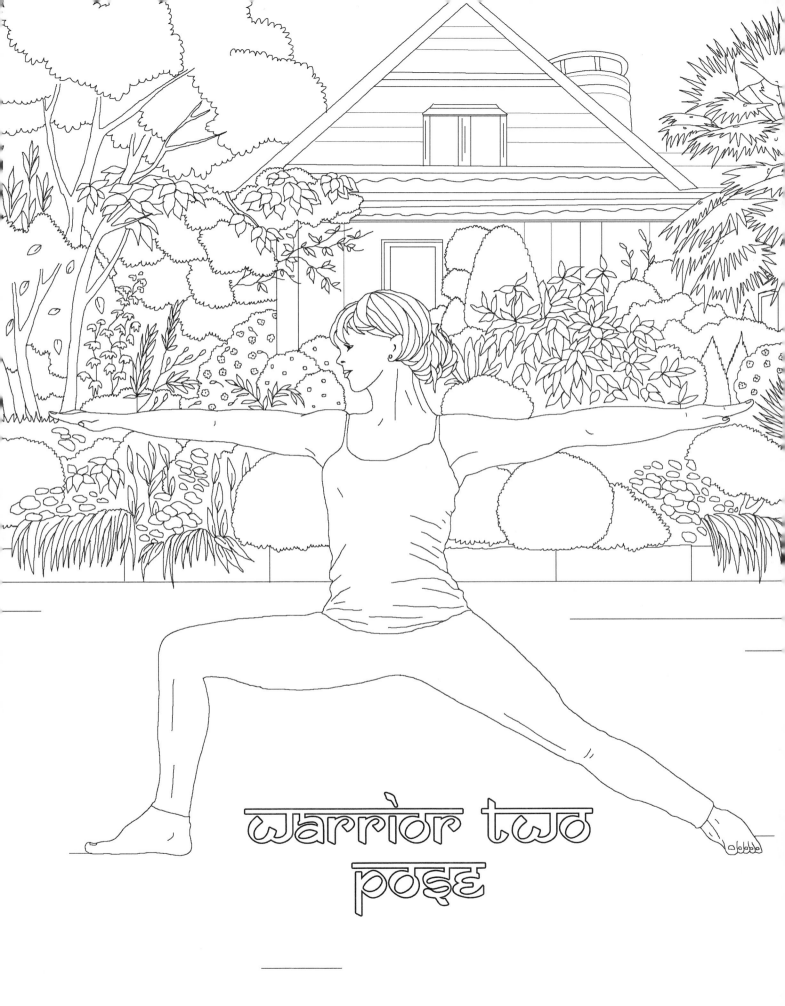

warrior two
pose

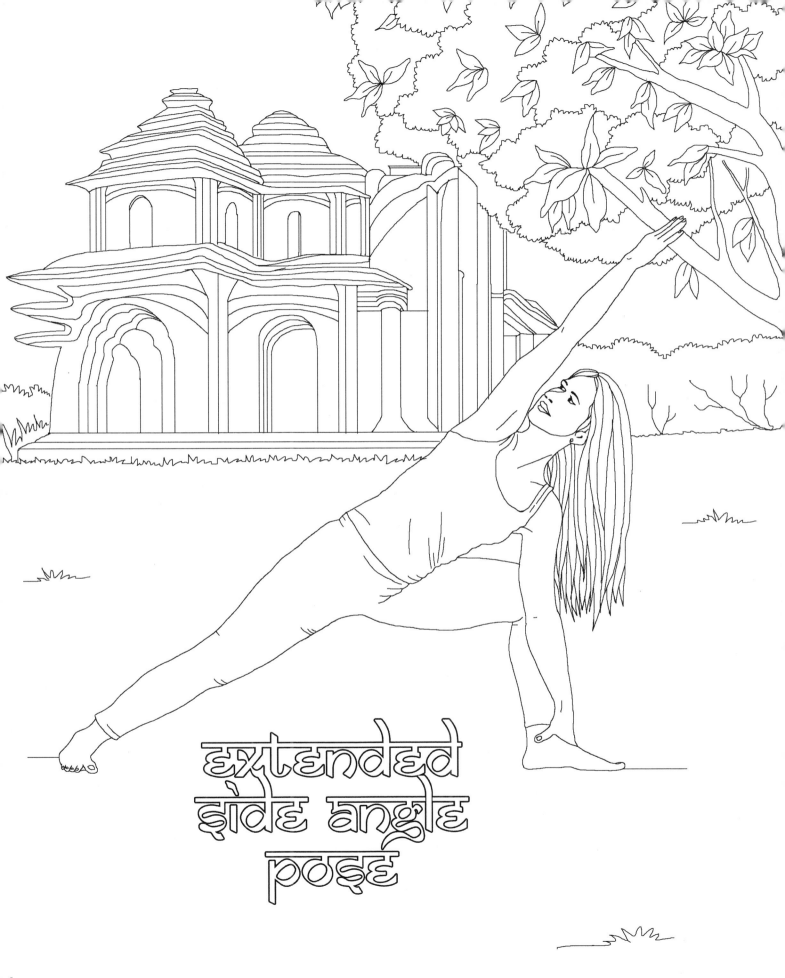

extended side angle pose

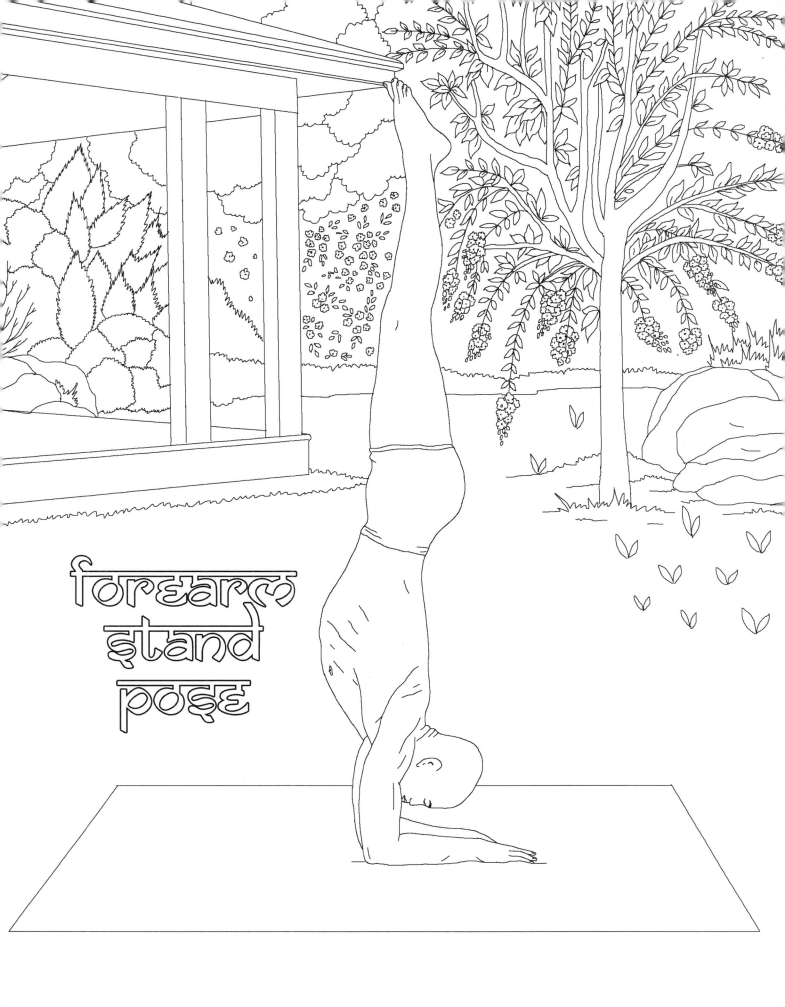

forearm
stand
pose

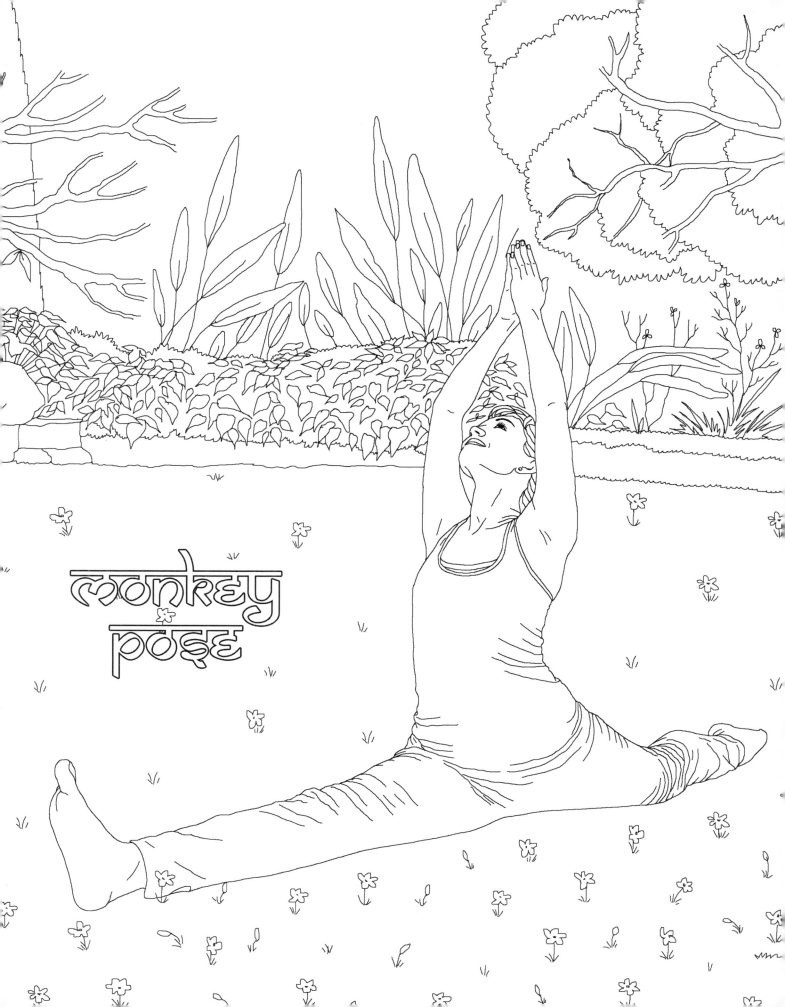

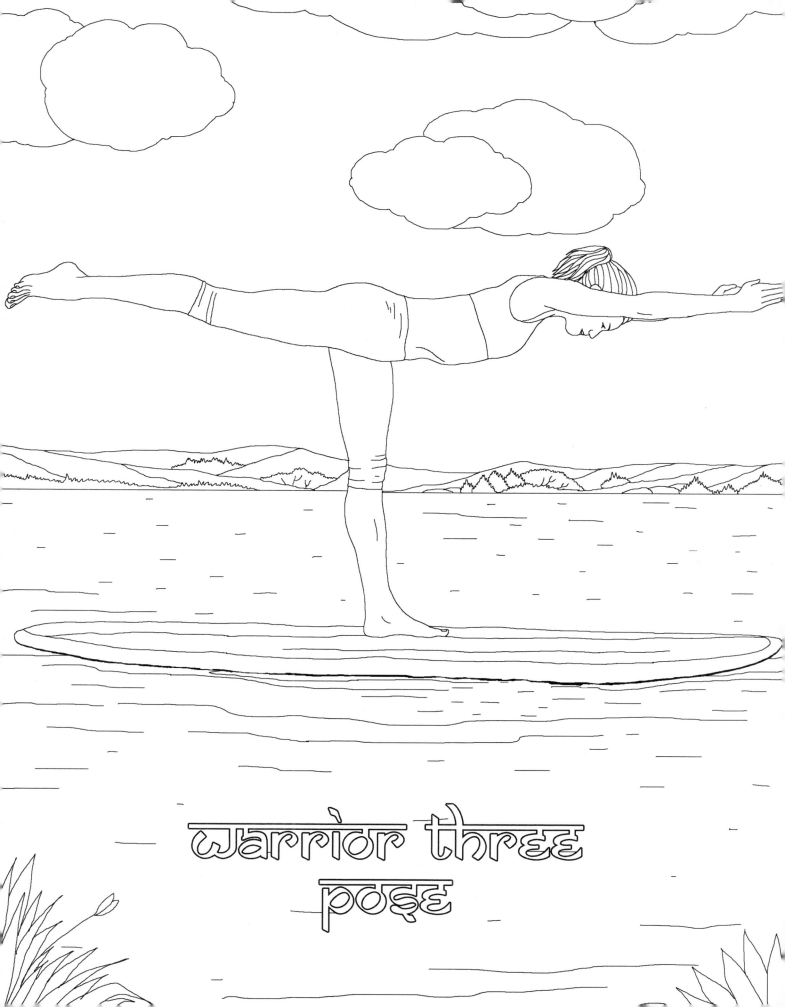

warrior three
pose

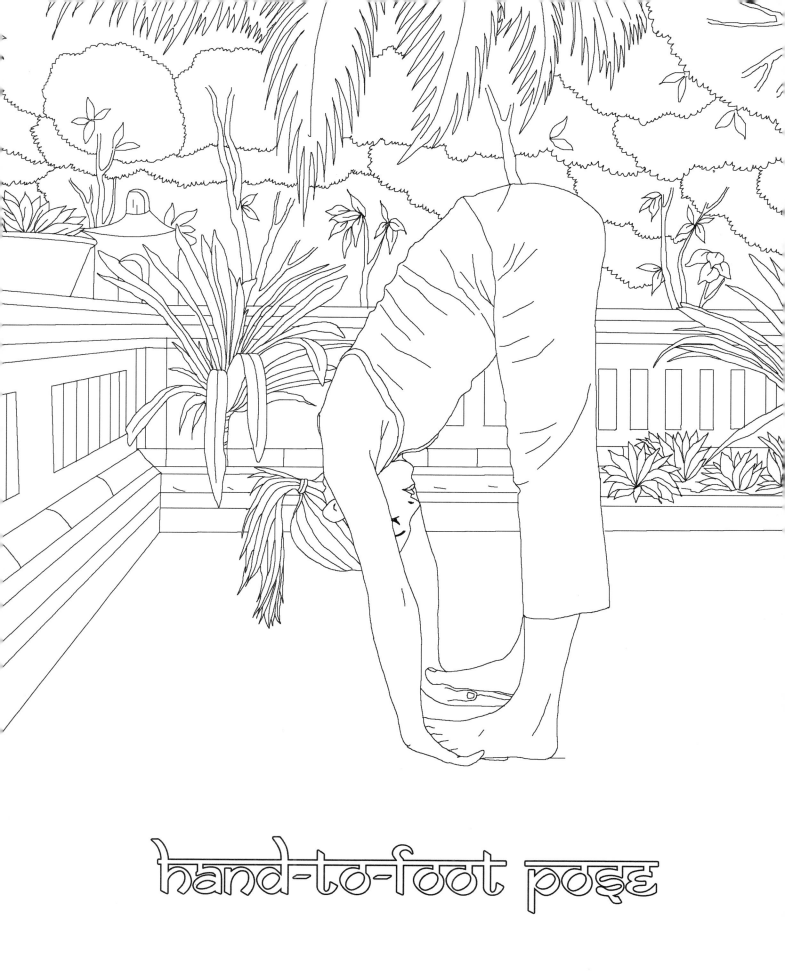

hand-to-foot pose

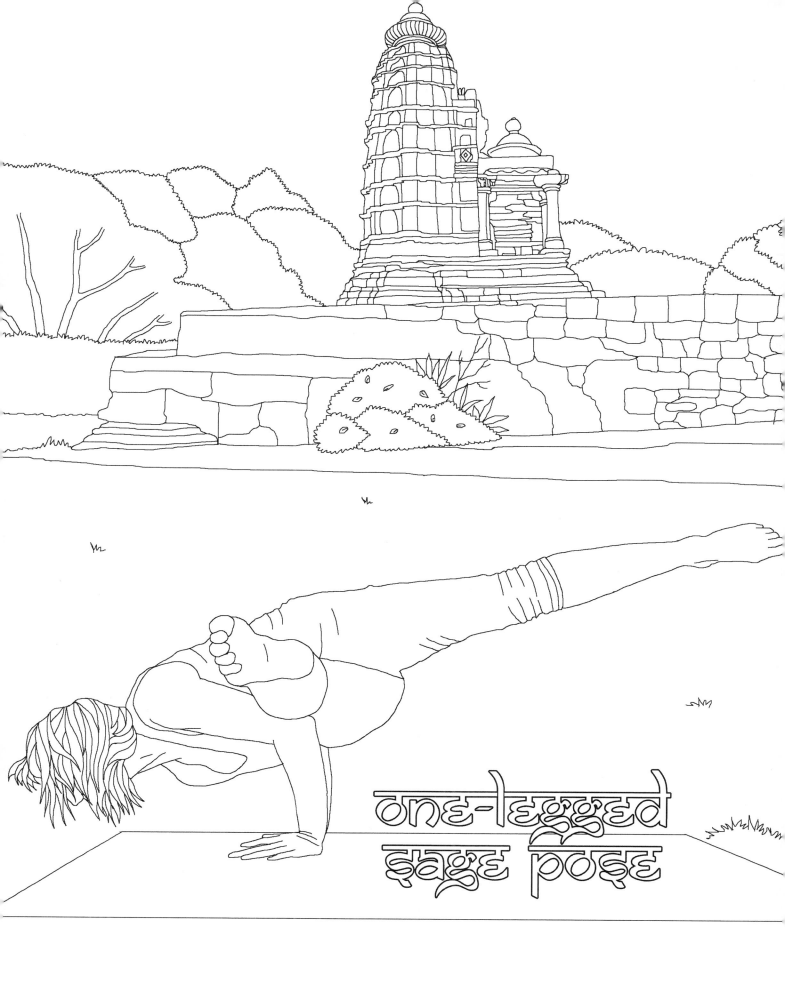

one-legged
sage pose

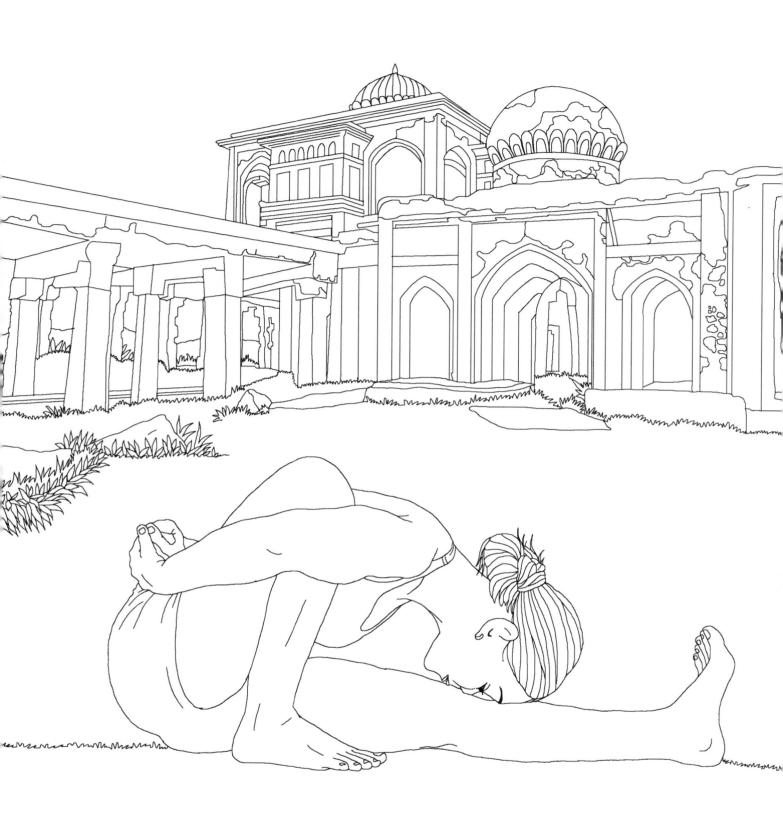

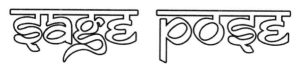

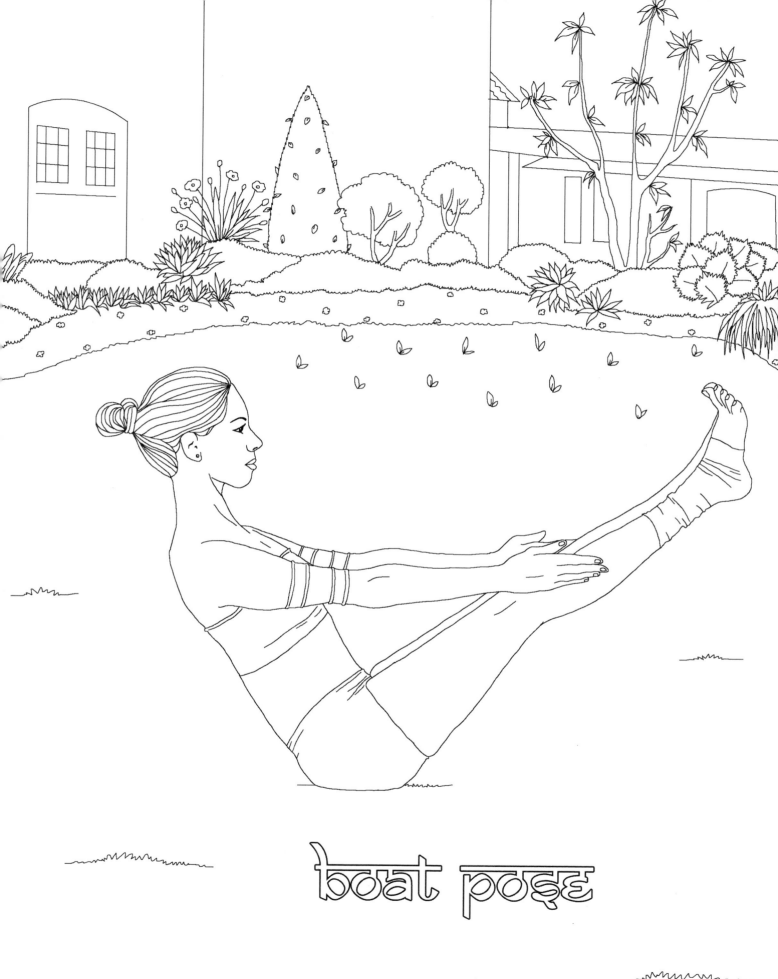

boat pose

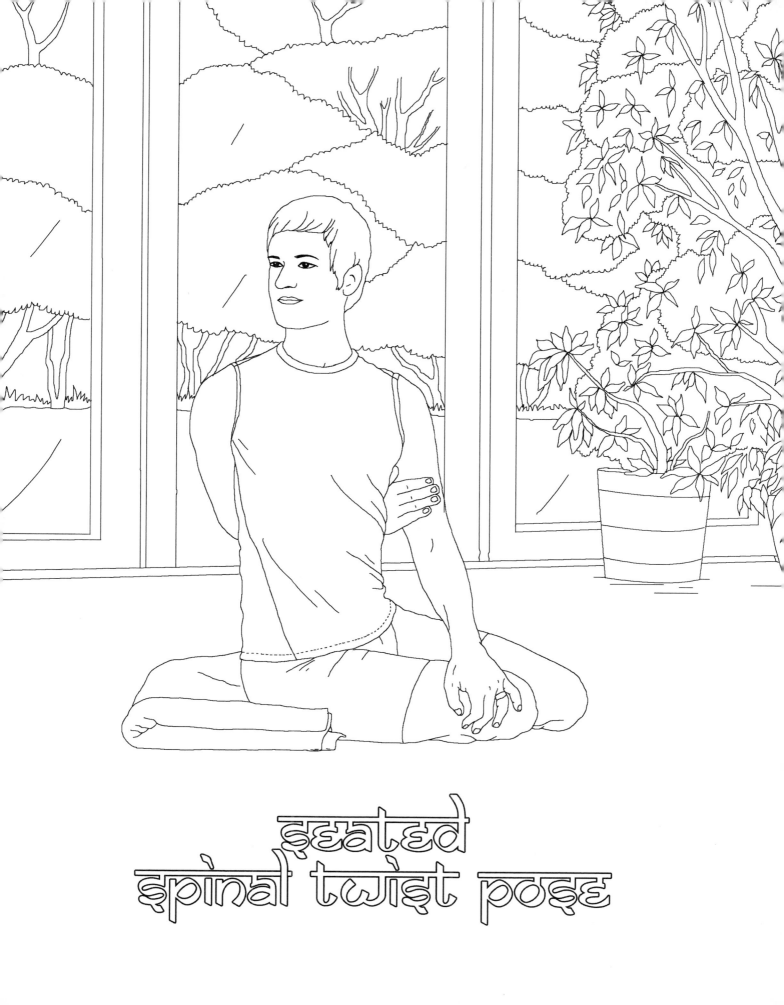

seated
spinal twist pose

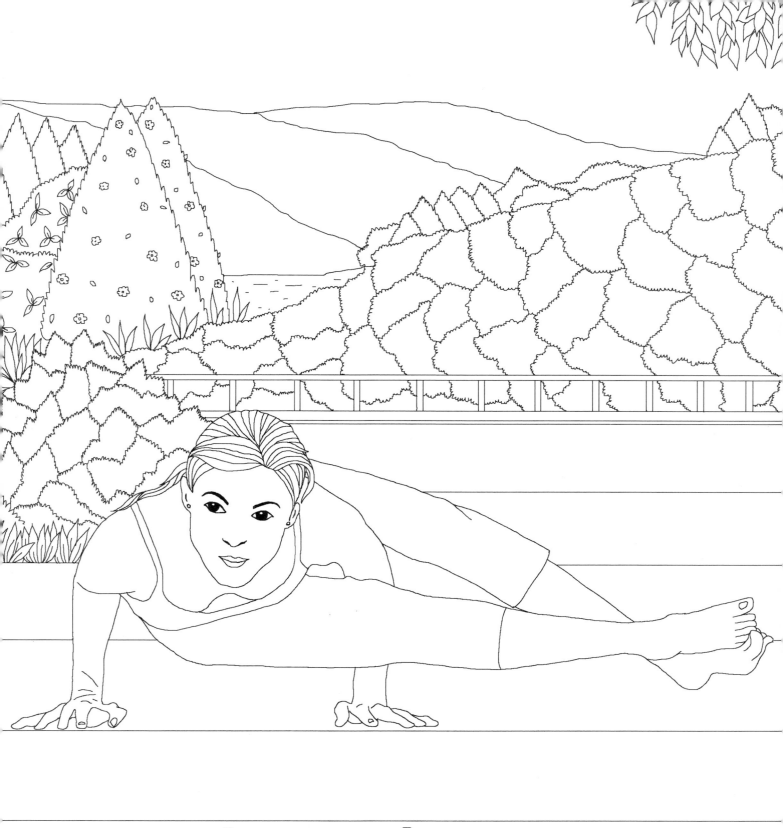

eight angle pose

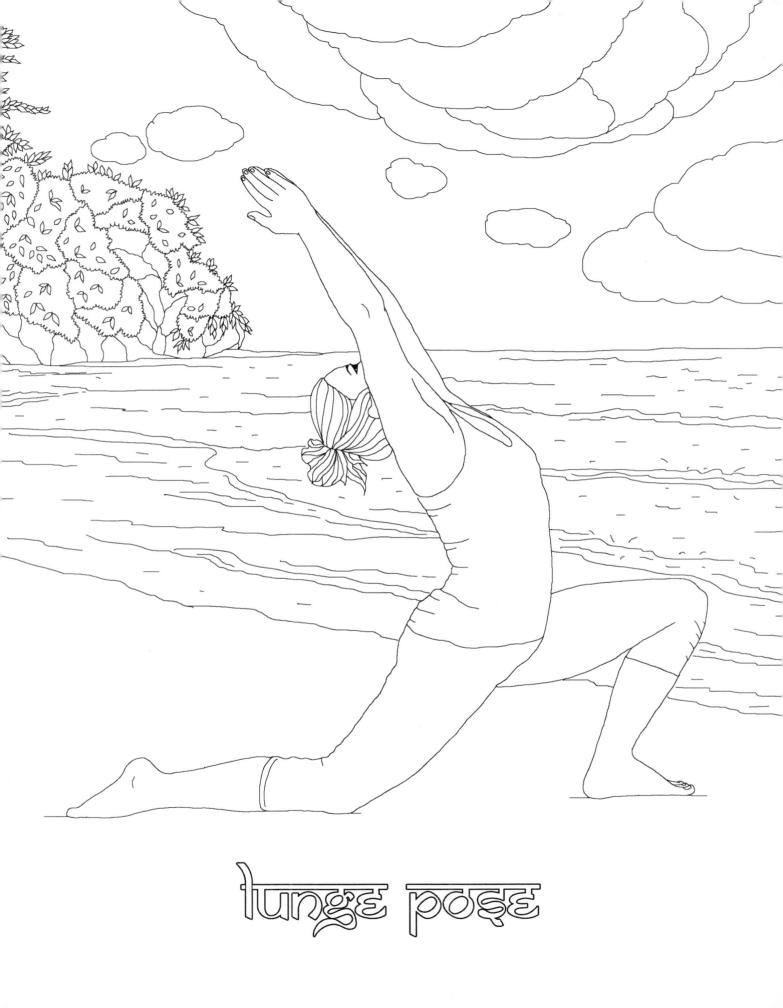

lunge pose

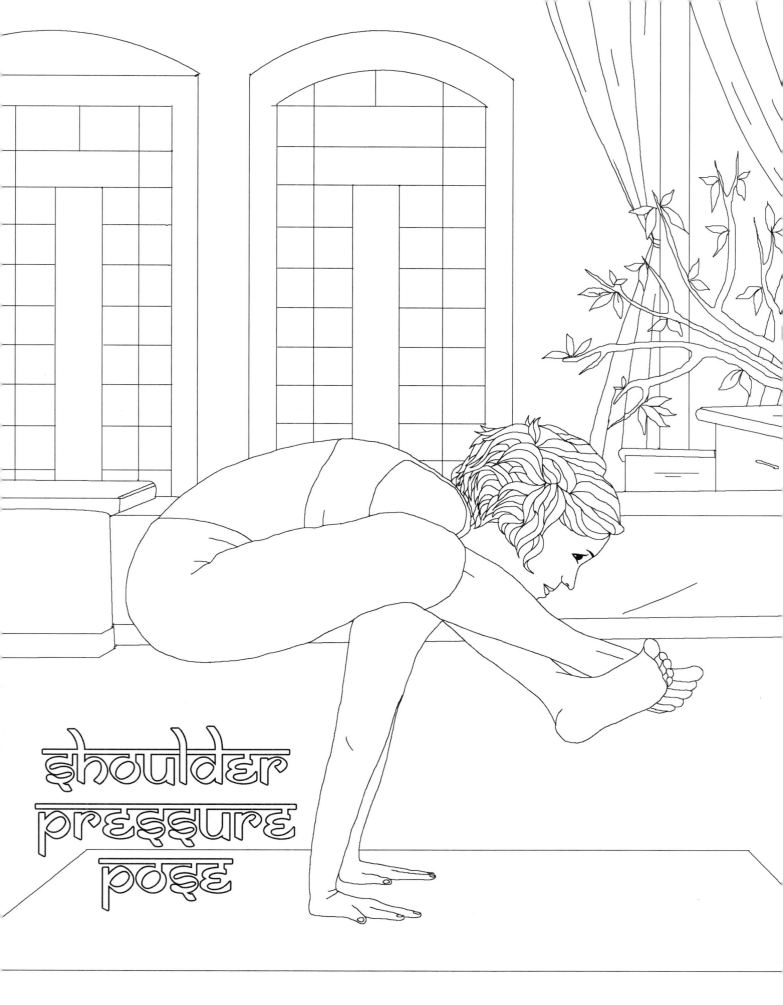

shoulder
pressure
pose

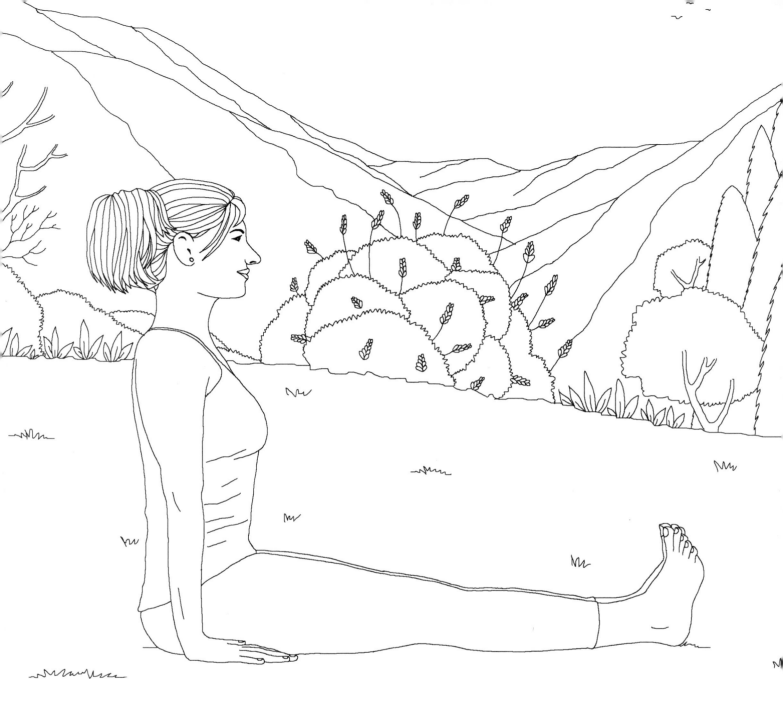

staff pose

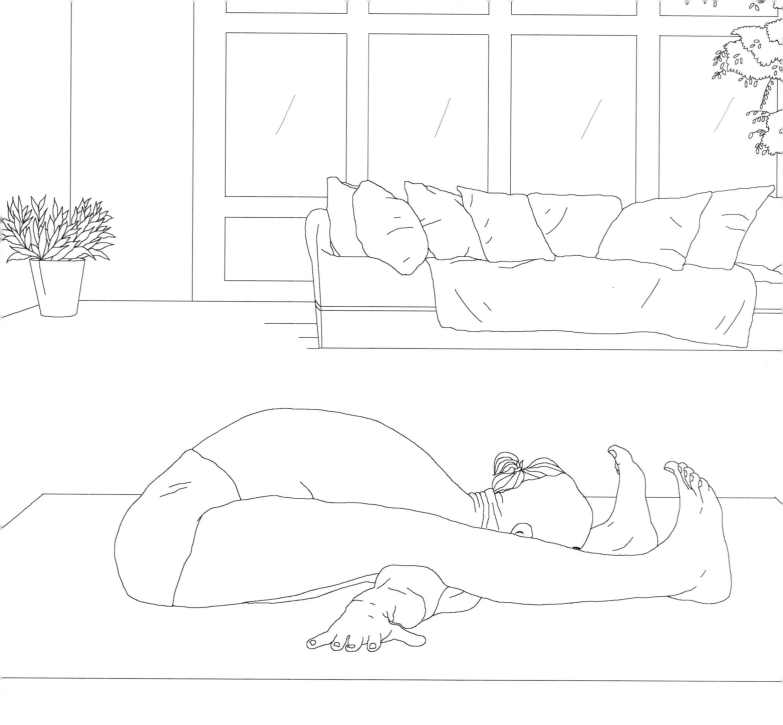

tortoise pose

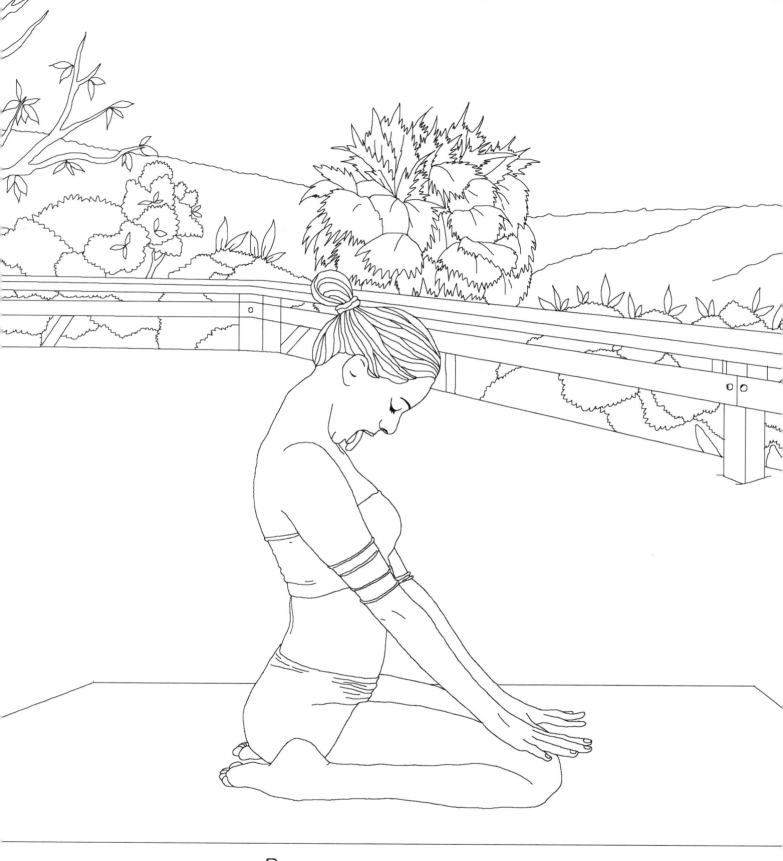

lion pose

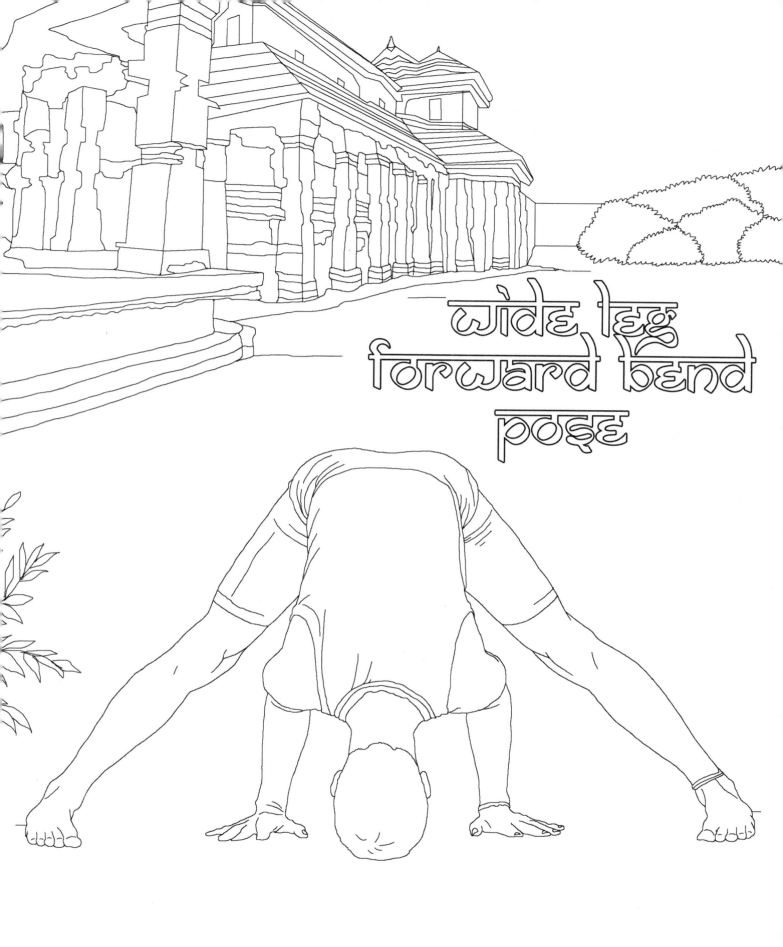

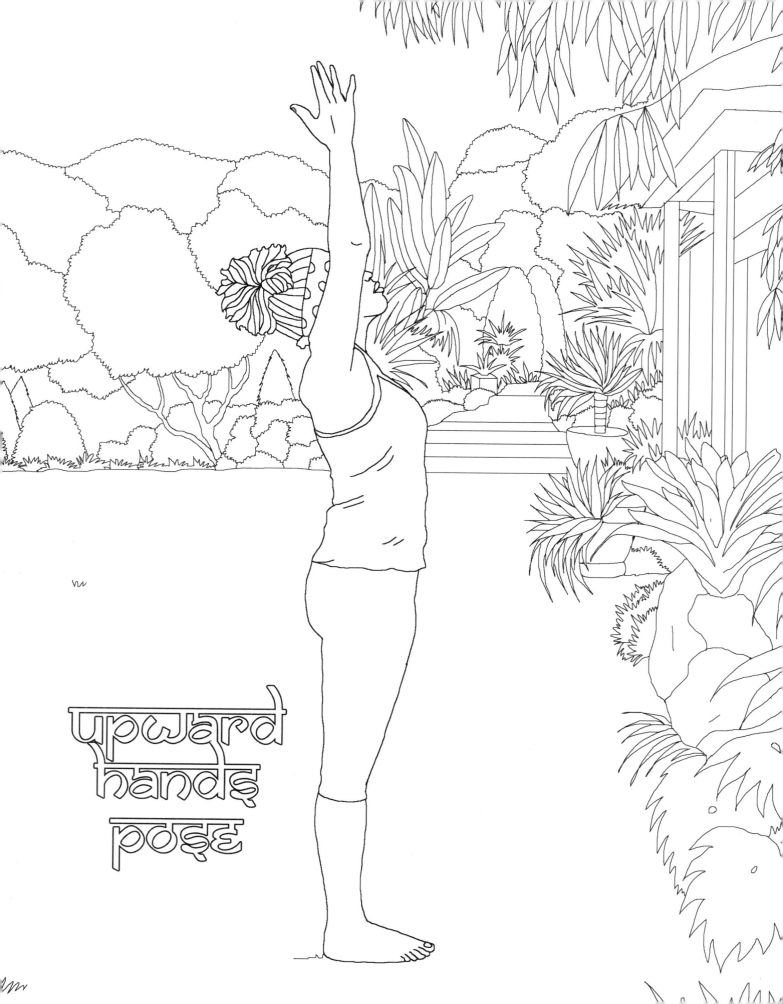

upward
hands
pose